Pregnancy & Childbirth Tips

Gail J. Dahl

To Lyn,
Best wishes,

Innovative Publishing
#2755, 349 West Georgia Street, Vancouver, BC, V6B 3X2
Email: innovative.publishing@shaw.wave.ca
Web Page: http://calgary.shaw.wave.ca/pregnancytips

Innovative Publishing
Copyright© 1998 Gail J. Dahl
Cover Design Copyright© 1998 Innovative Publishing
Innovative Publishing, Vancouver, Canada V6B 3X2
Email: pregnancy.tips@shaw.wave.ca

Canadian Cataloguing In Publication Data
Dahl, Gail J.
ISBN 1-896937-00-4

Tips on pregnancy, childbirth, breastfeeding & newborn care.
Includes Index, Bibliography and Childbirth Resource Directory.
1. Pregnancy-Popular works. 2. Childbirth-Popular works.
3. Infant (Newborn)-Care. 4. Breastfeeding 5. Mother and Infant
RG525.D34 1998   618.2   C98-910356-5

Printed In Canada   10 9 8 7 6 5 4 3 2 1

Single copies may be ordered directly from the publisher.
A discount will be automatically assigned to any
purchase of five books and over.

*This book is dedicated to my daughter Jade,
my inspiration and anchor,
so that your world might be different.*

Pregnancy & Childbirth Tips

Gail J. Dahl

Contents

Chapter 1 – First Month 1
Calculating Your Due Date
Prenatal Vitamins
Preventing Birth Defects
Natural Remedies for Morning Sickness
Choosing Your Health Team
What You Need to Know Before You Have Your Baby:
    Choosing a Good Birth Practitioner

Chapter 2 – Second Month 9
Prenatal Visits
Personal Birth Plan
Amniocentesis & Chorionic Villus Sampling
Midwives & Doulas
What You Need to Know Before You Have Your Baby:
    What You Can Do To Prevent Premature Birth

Chapter 3 – Third Month 23
Connecting With Your Baby
Natural Remedies for High Blood Pressure
Natural Remedies for Constipation
Health Risks of Tobacco, Drugs and Alcohol During Pregnancy
Leading New Discoveries on Nutrition During Pregnancy
What You Need to Know Before You Have Your Baby:
    Electronic Monitoring Devices – Why You Don't Need Them
    Drugs During Labor and Delivery – Is Any Drug Safe?
    Ultrasound – Valid Test or Smoke & Mirrors?

Chapter 4 – Fourth Month 37
The Woman's Herb
Exercising
Breastfeeding Facts
Breastfeeding Secrets
What You Need to Know Before You Have Your Baby:
    Breech Presentation – Medical Fashion Changes
    Gestational Diabetes – Fact or Fiction?
    Rupture of Membranes – New Answers

Chapter 5 – Fifth Month 49
Managing Fear of Labor and Delivery
The Wise Women
What You Need to Know Before You Have Your Baby:

Preventing Episiotomy
Birth Inductions – Unsafe at Any Speed

Acknowledgments

To the more than fifty professionals, physicians, midwives, homeopaths, registered nurses, professional labor support people, doulas, prenatal educators and instructors, breastfeeding specialists, newborn caregivers, childbirth researchers and educators who reviewed and commented on this guide and who contributed their uniquely feminine point of view, both personally and professionally, I give my heartfelt thanks.

I would also like to thank the following people for their excellent support and contributions to the project. Thanks to the others not listed who also gave of their time, ideas, and energy to help make this project happen. This book has become a tapestry, brilliantly woven through, with the love that women have for one another.

Abraham, Margaret	Abraham, Valerie
Abrahamson, Cheryl	Allyjan, Arlette
Anderson, Kari	Andersons, Mar
Apassin, Shirley	Apfield, Lisa
Babin, Kimberly	Baker, Jane
Beck, Janine	Begley, Sharon
Berg, Lily	Berreth, Selina
Bishop, Daphne	Blasetti, Karen
Boettcher, Monica	Boles, Franka
Bowen, Melanie	Brouwers, Nicole
Bruce, Deanna	Campbell, Jo-Anne
Chovancak, Beata	Colecallough, Kathleen
Collins, Bridget	Cohen, Nancy Wainer
Comito, Rosa	Cross, Maureen
Cuttrill, Linda	Dahl, Chelsea
Dahl, Kathy	Dahl, Nola
Dahl, Martin	Day, Sarah
Debiche, Dorothy	Debott, Iris
DeMarco, Carolyn	Devetten, Linda
Dinsmore, Katherine	Dobson, Rosemary
Dorosh, Natasha	Doucette, Dori Gallelli
Dubrick, Kathryn	Duffee, Sonya
Dusang, Tanya	Edwards, Julie
Eichhorst, Shelley	Eschpeter, Colleen
Estner, Lois	Elliot, Grace
Farris, Lois	Fink, Kimberley
Flaig, Kim	Fordyce, Patricia
Fox, Rebecca	Fraser, Bobbie
Galas, Ula	Gardy, Ernie
Gardy, Jade	Gilhooly, Kathleen
Gillespie, Christine	Giroux, Janis

Goer, Henci
Goulet, Laura
Grandy, Charlotte
Grant, Denise
Greene, Vanecea
Halls, Anita
Harper, Carol
Harries, Sandra
Henderson, Therese
Hernandez, Tina
Hill, Angie
Holnus, Dorothy
Huculak, Elaine
Isabella, Melanie
Janissen, Marlene
Johnson, Christie
Johnston, Marion
Jones, Louise
Kardal, Lori
Kitzinger, Sheila
Kovach, Sylvie
Lawson, Darcy
Lefebrre, Kathy
Lemke, Andy
Loewen, Michelle
Luke, Barbara
Lyon, Iris
Macdonald, Anne
Manuel, Barb
Marsh, Kim
McKeage, Wendy
Melling, Helen
Mikkelson, Fay
Moulton, Meryl
Nagy-Cherrett, Heather
Nation, Barbara
Nightingale, Joanna
Patterson, Mrs.
Place, Kelly
Poppleton, Sharon
Priaulx, Tina
Randall, Kim
Reid, Catherine

Golant, Susan
Gourley, Gwynneth
Graham, Janis
Greene, Aeriol
Griffin, Nancy
Harms, Jamie
Harper, Michelle
Helenka, Lauren
Herkert, Kimberly Ann
Hibberd, Justine
Hill, Nadia
Honard, Lynne
Hurley, Janette
Jacobsen, Gloria
Jessmaine, Cheryl
Johnston, Cheryl
Joncas, Leanne
Kabtiymer, Zenebech
Kenrick, Mariam
Kolibar, Shelley
Lamb, Lynn
Leach, Penelope
Leibel, Dee
Lindstrom, Denise
Ludington-Hoe, Susan
Luxford, Joy
MacAusland, Margaret
MacDonald, Colette
Merricks, Cathy
McKay, Margaret
McPhee, Paula
Milne, Vivian
Morales, Karla
Mulanson, Lisa
Nason, Zoria
Nicholls, Debbie
O'Neil, Melody
Picketts, Helene
Placksin, Sally
Pratt, Jodi
Raby-Dunne, Susan
Raymond, Kitty
Rehlinger, Lucy

Rod, Susan
Saint, Emilia
Sandwell, Jollean
Serhan, Nancy
Sewyl, Francine
Sinanon, Stephanie
Smythe, Angela
Spooner, Cindy
St.Pierre, Shawna
Skyllard, Rose
Taylor, Rachael
Vestrum, Tammy
Warner, Kim
Wiebe, Joy
Willson, Sharon
Winters, Staci
Young, Robin

Rychyk, Rose
Sanche, Cynthia
Scarlett, Sheila
Sethi, Sarla
Shepard, Trish
Sinclair, Lee
Sonnenberg, Carol
Stech, Brenda
Stevens, Dave
Szrubec, Barb
Turner, Karen
Wallach, Joel
West, Joy
Williams, Delane
Wilson, Lynn
Young, Catherine

INTRODUCTION

As I started out on the incredible journey of bringing in a new life, I searched for information that would guide me safely to this next destination. I remember throwing the last book across the room wondering why it was so difficult to find information on what really happened during the birth process. I wanted to read what other mothers had discovered through their own practical experience and to learn from them. I also wanted to be informed of the newest scientific discoveries on childbirth.

During my research, I discovered that many of today's mothers have opted out of the typical assembly-line birth plan offered by many of the hospitals and are reclaiming this powerful experience for themselves by choosing to have their next children with the assistance of professional labor support. They had choreographed every detail of the birth of their baby like a play or a movie, creating the script (your birth plan), hiring the actors (creating your health team), directing the support people, as well as having the starring role. Many women had created an excellent health support team to guide them through the birth process and beyond.

Some women I interviewed had difficult experiences and wanted to pass on their information to help other women have an easier and safer birth. In the end, I was surprised to find out that many of today's common medical interventions, like IVs, drugs, epidurals, having to labor on your back, endless mechanical fetal monitoring, routine episiotomy, being unable to eat or drink to keep your strength up during labor or the routine use of drugs to force or speed up labor, can actually cause your labor to become more painful and prolonged and your baby's delivery more difficult. Mounting evidence is showing that each needless birth intervention puts the mother and baby at an ever increasing risk of complications. Take the time to investigate the risks and side effects that these common medical interventions can have on you and your baby. In some circumstances, some of the time, some medical interventions are necessary. Informed consent and knowledge of your natural birth process will assist you in evaluating each medical intervention on its own merit in consultation with the health team you have assembled.

In this pregnancy guide you will find information on preventing premature birth, natural remedies for common pregnancy problems, the value of hiring professional labor support, and watching and waiting as an alternative to forcing labor. You will read about new effective pain relief during labor, tips on assisting your baby to descend faster, midwive's techniques for moving stalled labor, how to have a faster, easier and safer delivery along with other leading new research that will assist you in making informed, intelligent decisions regarding the health of you and your baby.

The Childbirth Resource Directory has been included to guide you to the best prenatal and postnatal services in your city. Researchers from around the world have contributed vital information that you need to know before you have your baby. Mothers of every age have contributed their practical knowledge and experience on pregnancy, childbirth, breastfeeding and newborn care. The recommended reading list will guide you in locating some of the best pregnancy and childbirth books for further study.

Birth is a normal, natural, empowering experience. Studies are showing that more than 95% of women are capable of giving birth without any help or interference. Women around the world are reclaiming this empowering experience by choosing to birth with women and with those who are experienced with normal, natural birth. This guidebook is like having your grandmother, mother, sister and friends in attendance to give you the emotional, physical, spiritual and intellectual support that was once easily available through our community of family and friends.

May this book guide you and give you the confidence to enjoy every stage of your birth process and lead you to a safe and satisfying childbirth for you and your baby.

Best wishes, Gail J. Dahl

CHILDBIRTH RESOURCE DIRECTORY
CANADA

To assemble your health team in Canada, contact your local Childbirth Association or Midwife Association for referrals on the best birth physicians, birth clinics, independent midwives, nurse-midwives, doulas, professional labor support assistants, prenatal instructors and classes, lactation consultants, breastfeeding groups and postnatal support in your city. Childbirth Associations and Midwife Associations are not-for-profit groups and are staffed by volunteer parents and professionals who are there to help you design the best birth for you and your baby.

BRITISH COLUMBIA

Pacific Prenatal Education Association
PO Box 3059, Mission, V2V 4J3 (604) 467-4259
Vaginal Birth After Cesarean
4006 Nithdale Street, Burnaby, V5G 1P6 (604) 433-5827
Vancouver Childbirth Association
4340 Carson, Burnaby (604) 437-9968
Midwives Association of British Columbia
#55, 2147 Commercial Drive, Vancouver, V5N 5B3 (604) 736-5976
Midwifery Task Force of British Columbia
PO Box 65343, Station F, Vancouver, (604) 251-5976
College of Midwives of British Columbia
#F502, 4500 Oak Street, Vancouver, V6H 3N1 (604) 875-3580
Vancouver Women's Health Collective
219, 1675 W. Eighth Avenue, Vancouver, V6J 1V2 (604) 736-4234
Founded to promote women's active participation in and control of their own health care. Information is available on postpartum depression, birthing options, local support groups and more. They also maintain a health practitioner directory with notes from women evaluating the care they have received from individual health practitioners in the city.
Vancouver Breastfeeding Center
690 West 11th Avenue, Vancouver, V5Z lMl (604) 875-4730
The center offers prenatal lactation assessments, anticipatory guidance and early intervention strategies as well as a variety of training courses for health professionals.
Pacific Post Partum Support Society
104, 1416 Commercial Drive, Vancouver, V5L 3X9 (604) 255-7999
Offers weekly support groups, telephone counselling and information nights for fathers.

ALBERTA

Calgary Association of Parents and Professionals for Safe Alternatives in Childbirth, CAPSAC

300, 223 – 12th Avenue SW, Calgary, T2R OG9 (403) 237-8839

Providing safe, family-centered maternal and newborn programs to meet the social and emotional needs of women and their families based on informed choices in childbirth.

Association for Safe Alternatives in Childbirth, ASAC

203, 9924 – 106 Street, Edmonton, T5J 2M4 (403) 425-7993

A consumer group concerned with choices in childbirth.

Peace River Childbirth Education Association

11417 – 103 Street, Peace River, T8S lL9 (403) 624-2623

Alberta Association of Midwives

PO Box 1705, Main Post Office, Edmonton, T5J 2P1 (403) 435-6278

Midwifery Consumers of Alberta Network

Box 401, Black Diamond TOL OHO (403) 933-7204

Vaginal Birth After Cesarean

8403-77 Street, Edmonton, T6C 2L7 (403) 465-2822

Briar Hill Birth Center – Free Standing Birth Clinic

1616 20A Street NW, Calgary, T2N 2L5 (403) 289-8334

The Birth Place – Free Standing Birth Clinic

5415 – 49th Avenue, Red Deer, T4N 3X5 (403) 342-4661

Kensington Family Health Clinic

1167 Kensington Cres. NW, Calgary, T2N lX7 (403)270-0440

A team of physicians, midwives, prenatal instructors, and lactation consultants.

Canadian Lactation Consultant Association

852 Knottwood Road S., Edmonton, T6K 3C3 (403) 462-1848

A professional association of breastfeeding consultants across Canada.

Calgary Breastfeeding Clinic

1616 – 20A Street NW, Calgary, T2N 2L5 (403) 242-4205

Offers classes for parents and consultation for mothers having difficulties as well as educational programs for health professionals.

Infant Resource Center

2531 – 25 Avenue SW Calgary, T3E OK1 (403) 242-3533

Offers support and education to new parents. Offers classes and discussion groups on sleeping problems, discipline, toilet training and other topics of interest.

The Family Center

20, 9912-106 Street, Edmonton, T5K 1C5 (403) 423-2831

This center is staffed by more than 200 professionals and volunteers and offers a wide spectrum of support services to families using a subsidized fee structure. Services include homemakers, workshops on all aspects of parenting, home support for new mothers, and a postpartum depression program.

The Postpartum Depression Support Program
20, 9912 106th Street, Edmonton, T5K 1C5 (403) 423-2831
Offers telephone contact, home visits, weekly group meetings and other helpful services.

Calgary Post Partum Support Society
405 – 52nd Avenue SW, Calgary, T2V OB1 (403) 253-6722
Offers moms a telephone match with a carefully trained and selected volunteer who has experienced and resolved postpartum depression.

Calgary Family Connections Society
6305 – 33 Avenue NW, Calgary, (403) 288-8111
Offers a free Toy Lending Library and provides educational and emotional support for families with a view to long-term academic and social success for children.

Parents and Children Together (403) 252-2211
A fun playful environment for parents and children. Discussion topics include parenting styles, communication, child development, coping with temper tantrums, effective discipline for preschoolers and understanding self-esteem. Nine locations throughout Calgary.

SASKATCHEWAN

Midwives Association of Saskatchewan
312 Main Street, Saskatoon, S7N OB7 (306) 653-1349

Friends of the Midwives
3223 McCallum Ave, Regina, S4S OR7 (306) 586-6441
512 9th St. East, Saskatoon, S7N OB1 (306) 652-4289

Midwifery Practices in Saskatchewan
2210 Athol Street, Regina, S4T 3E9 (306) 586-2241 or 585-1674
312 Main Street, Saskatoon, S7N OB7 (306) 653-1349 or 653-3755

MANITOBA

Association of Manitoba Midwives
PO Box 83, Norwood Post Office, Winnipeg, R2H 3B8 (204) 687-1960

Manitoba Home Birth Network
#5, 131 Tyndall Avenue, Winnipeg (204) 697-0574

Traditional Midwives of Manitoba Collective
487 Telfer Street South, Winnipeg, R3G 2Y4 (204) 775-3862

Women's Health Clinic

419 Graham Avenue, Winnipeg, R3C OM3 (204) 947-1517
Provides women-centered care in a variety of issues, including postpartum stress and offers a holistic and multifaceted approach in an atmosphere that is respectful, informative, compassionate and nonjudgemental.

QUEBEC
Quebec Midwives Alliance
CP246, Succ E., Montreal, H2T 3A7 (514) 278-8650
Association Des Sages-Femmes Du Quebec
Box 354, Station Cote-des-Neiges, Montreal, H3S 2S6 (514) 738-8090
Ligue Internationale La Leche Inc.
725, Rue Buchanan, St-Laurent, H4L 2T8
Center Local de Services Communautaires de la Haute-Yamaska
294 Deragon Street, Granby, J2G 5J5 (514) 375-1442
Nourri-Source
CP 441 Succ. Montreal Nord, H1H 5L5 (418) 663-2711

ONTARIO
Association of Ontario Midwives
#205, 2050 Sheppard Avenue E., North York, M2J 5B3 (416) 494-4819
Ontario Midwifery Consumer Network
260 Adelaide Street E, PO Box 64, Toronto (416) 767-0427
College of Midwives of Ontario
PO Box 2213, Station P – Suite 285, Toronto, M5S 2T2 (416) 658-8715
Vaginal Birth After Cesarean Canada
991 Glen Cairn Avenue, Toronto, M5N 1T8 (416) 489-7710
Friends of Breastfeeding Society
RR #2, Chesley, NOG lLO (519) 363-3778
La Leche League Canada
PO Box 29, 18C Industrial Drive, Chesterville, KOC 1HO (613) 448-1842
Call Toll Free For Your Neighborhood Meeting Location 1-800-665-4324
Informal meetings held monthly to discuss various aspects of breastfeeding. There is no charge for meetings or telephone consultations on any questions regarding breastfeeding your baby.
Family Service Canada
#600, 220 Laurier Avenue W, Ottawa, K1P 5Z9 (613) 230-9960
This non-profit group is associated with over one hundred agencies across Canada offering assistance with marital problems, parent-child difficulties, single parenthood and any other family related problems.
The Canadian Association of Toy Libraries and Parent Resource Center
205, 120 Holland Avenue, Ottawa, KlY OX6 (613) 728-3307

National organization offering parenting courses, peer support, child care services and toy libraries across Canada.

Toronto Women's Health Network

201, 489 College Street, Toronto, M6G 1A5

Educational and information sharing network based on the belief that women are their own experts with respect to their health care.

Women's Health Center

30 The Queensway, Toronto, M6R 1B5 (416) 530-6850

Offers a prenatal screening program, prenatal support program, maternal support classes, a program for postpartum depression and a multicultural health education program.

Childbirth Education Program with the Canadian Mothercraft Society

32 Heath Street W., Toronto, M4V 1T3 (416) 920-3515

A combination of seven prenatal and three postnatal classes. The postnatal classes are designed to ease the adjustment into parenting and to provide practical information and tips on infant care.

Moms Offering Mothers Support for Postnatal Depression

495 Richmond Road, Ottawa, K2A 4A4 (613) 722-2242

Offers weekly group meetings as well as regular telephone contact.

Not Just the Blues

Postpartum Adjustment Support Services

Box 7282, Oakville, L6J 6C6 (905) 844-9009

Provides individual, couple and parent-infant counselling, support group for mothers, support for fathers and a telephone buddy.

Mothers Are Women

PO Box 4104, Station E, Ottawa, K1S 5B1 (613) 722-7851

Concerned with the interests of women who have chosen to stay at home to raise their children. Provides monthly educational and experiential workshops on anger and guilt, self-esteem, money and power and career and life planning. Advocates for greater public and governmental awareness of the concerns of mothers at home.

MARITIMES

Association of Nova Scotia Midwives

PO Box 968, Wolfville, NS B0P 1XO (902) 582-3151

Vaginal Birth After Cesarean

Dariah Purdy, Yarmouth County, NS B0W 2VO

New Mothers Resource Group

Box 1271, Liverpool, NS B0T 1KO

New Brunswick Midwives Association

200 Inglewood Drive, Fredericton, NB E3B 2K6 (506) 459-3172
Breastfeeding Consultation Service
30 Avondale Drive, Riverview, NB E1B 1C2 (506) 386-6057
Alliance of Nurse-Midwives, Maternal and Pediatric Nurses
PO Box 8352, Station A, St. John's, NF A1B 3N7
Newfoundland and Labrador Midwives Association
c/o School of Nursing, Memorial University, St. John's, NF (709) 737-6577

YUKON AND THE NORTHWEST TERRITORIES
Midwives Association of British Columbia
#55, 2147 Commercial Drive, Vancouver, BC (604) 436-600

SAMPLE AREA
We have assembled the Directory to assist you with locating and assembling your own health team in your city. Here is a representative sample of the services available in the province of Alberta, Canada. To get the most current names of services, telephone numbers and addresses in your area, visit, write or telephone your local Childbirth Association or Midwives Association listed in the Childbirth Resource Directory. Let them know what you plan for the birth of your baby and they will assist you at no charge in locating the services you require. Always be prepared to interview a number of prospective health team members and to call references so that you feel completely comfortable with the service they offer.

ALBERTA, CANADA – CHILDBIRTH ASSOCIATIONS
Calgary Association of Parents and Professionals for Safe Alternatives in Childbirth (CAPSAC) (403) 237-8839 #300, 223 – 12th Avenue S.W. Calgary T2R OG9.
CAPSAC is dedicated to exploring, implementing and establishing safe, family-centered maternal and newborn programs that meet the social and emotional needs of women and their families as well as to provide safe, appropriate aspects of medical science based on informed choice. CAPSAC has an extensive lending library available to members and has sponsored childbirth conferences and speakers. Meetings are held on the third Wednesday of each month, members and non-members welcome. CAPSAC keeps a up-to-date directory of birth services offered in the city of Calgary, Alberta and in the surrounding communities and publishes the internationally known magazine "Birth Issues".
Association for Safe Alternatives in Childbirth, (ASAC), (403) 425-7993 P.O. Box 1197, Main Post Office, #203, 9924 – 106 Street, Edmonton T5J 2M4.
ASAC is a consumer group concerned with choices in childbirth.

Peace River Childbirth Education Association (403) 624-2623
11417 – 103 Street, Peace River, T8S lL9
The Alberta Association of Midwives (403) 289-8334
1616 – 20A Street NW, Calgary, T2N 2L5
Midwifery Consumers of Alberta Network (MCAN) 933-7204
Box 401, Black Diamond, TOL OHO
VBAC – Vaginal Birth After Cesarean (403) 465-2822
8403-77 Street, Edmonton, T6C 2L7

FREE-STANDING BIRTH CLINICS
Briar Hill Birth Center (403) 289-8334
1616 – 20A Street NW, Calgary, T2N 2L5
The Birth Place (403) 342-4661
5415 – 49th Avenue, Red Deer, T4N 3X5

MIDWIFE TEAMS
Edmonton and Area Independently Practicing Midwives
Damsma, Annita – With Woman Midwifery 425-0916
Ellis, Maureen – Birth Choices Midwifery 413-6142
Flanagan, Kerstin – Passages Midwifery 431-0181
Gibbons, Donna – Gibbons & Tutt 413-8982
Gostkowski, Martha – Natural Birth 439-3200
Greenhalgh, Joanna – Birth Choices Midwifery 413-6142
James, Susan – With Woman Midwifery 425-0916
Lester, Wendy – Passages Midwifery 431-0181
Moore, Linda – Passages Midwifery 431-0181
Pullin, Sandy – With Woman Midwifery 425-0916
Scriver, Barbara – Passages Midwifery 431-0181
Tutt, Marie – Gibbons & Tutt 413-8982
Walker, Noreen – Passages Midwifery 431-0181
Calgary and Area Independently Practicing Midwives
Allyjan, Arlette – The Birth Partnership 246-8845
Day, Sara – Birth Wise Midwifery 276-2355
Dowell, Susan – Midwifery Collective 270-0440
Fraser, Bobbie – The Birth Partnership 246-8845
Galbraith, Kathy – Heartsongs 756-3013
Harvey, Sheila – The Birth Partnership 246-8845
Lenstra, Patty – Calgary & District Midwifery 289-8334
Moulton, Meryl – Calgary & District Midwifery 289-8334
Pettersson, Jo – Canmore Midwifery 678-6009
Robb, Karen – Birth Wise Midwifery 276-2355

Salkeld, Penny – Calgary & District Midwifery 289-8334
Smulders, Evonne – Midwifery Collective 270-0440
West, Joy – Calgary & District Midwifery 289-8334
Red Deer and Area Independently Practicing Midwives
Bacon, Joanna – Midwives Collective 347-8989
Fraser, Sharyne – The Birth Place 342-4661
Gajek, Trinda – The Birth Place 342-4661
MacDonald, Lize – Midwives Collective 347-8989
Purpur, Cherilynn – The Birth Place 342-4661
Welsh, Patricia – Midwives Collective 347-8989

DOULAS

Doula Services Association of Alberta (403) 590-0819
Kindred Spirits (403) 276-3760
Gaia Essences Corporation (403) 988-9217
Candice Gibson (403) 590-1366
Maureen Burghardt (403) 247-2947
Gwenyth Juric (403) 963-7991
Cathy Marricks (403) 640-2381
Elaine Montgomery (403) 252-4683
Nadine Hassen (403) 276-2355
Carolyn Johnston (403) 277-5370
Mary Van Woerkom (403) 295-2689
Rosemary Dobson (403) 686-1948
Debbie Tancsa (403) 569-9613
Lynette Hackey (403) 248-1539

PROFESSIONAL BIRTH ASSISTANTS

Sage Femme Maternity Services (403) 437-0676
Lia Berry (403) 228-7937
Loving Hands Labor Support (403) 464-7622
Joanne Gordon (403) 340-0820

PRENATAL CLASSES

Positive Birthing and Beyond (403) 288-3969 or 932-3978
The Bradley Method of Natural Childbirth (403) 258-1005
Joy Spring Childbirth Preparation (403) 464-2893
Calgary Immigrant Women's Association (403) 263-4414
Calgary Childbirth Education Association (403) 281-9485
New Beginnings (403) 449-4158
Beginnings Wholistic Health Services (403) 963-7991

BREASTFEEDING CLINICS AND CONSULTANTS

Calgary Breastfeeding Clinics (403) 242-4205
Birth and Breastfeeding Resources (403) 229-2522
La Leche League 1-800-665-4324 24 Hour Help Line
La Leche League (403) 242-0277 Calgary
Breastfeeding Clinic Lakeview (403) 246-7076
Nursing Mother's Support Group (403) 938-2707

POSTNATAL ASSISTANCE

Postnatal Helpers (403) 640-0844 (403) 459-8436
Calgary Community Support for Young Parents (403) 244-4040
The Primal Parenting Awareness Centre e:mail (nurturing@kjsl.com)
University of Calgary Prenatal & Postnatal Fitness (403) 220-5195
Postpartum Support (403) 253-6722
Infant Resource Center (403) 242-3533
Parent Development Resource Center (403) 253-6663
Calgary Family Connection Toy Lending Library (403) 288-8111
Calgary Learning Centre – Special Needs Children (403) 686-9300
City-Wide Time Out Groups (403) 286-5853
Early-Start Support for Families with New Babies 1-800-756-BABY
Foothills Support for Young Parents (4033) 244-4040
The Jellybean Tree – Special Needs Children (403) 241-0556
Jewish Family Services (403) 287-3510
Our Mother Earth Native Family Day Program (403) 240-4642
One-on-One Parent Education Service (403) 278-3145
Parent/Child Resource Consulting Group (403) 543-7580
Partners in Parenting (403) 225-0047
Providence Childrens' Center (403) 255-5577
Weavers Partnership of Family Life Educators (403) 284-1582
Whole Family Attachment Parenting Association (403) 247-1208

LOCAL PUBLICATIONS

Birth Issues #300, 223 – 12th Avenue S.W., Calgary (403) 237-883
Alberta Parent 248, 340-39th Avenue SE, Calgary (403) 243-8001
Nurturing Magazine #373, 918 – 16th Avenue NW Calgary T2M OK3 (403) 870-4005
The Western Parent 205, 1039 – 17 Avenue SW Calgary T2T OB2 (403) 543-3775
Calgary's Child 1008-246 Stewart Green SW Calgary T3H 3C8 (403) 520-1003

ADOPTION

Adoption by Choice (403) 245-8854
Adoption Options (403) 270-8228
Adoption Resource Foundation of Calgary (403) 276-9907
Adoption Services Crossroads Counselling (403)243-7876 (403)327-7080
Adoptive Counselling Calgary Family Service (403) 233-2370
Adoptive Parents Association (403) 278-3288

ALTERNATIVE HEALTH SERVICES

Kensington Family Health Clinic (403) 270-0440 Calgary.
A team of Family Physicians, Lactation Consultants, Midwives and Prenatal Instructors
Healing Arts (403) 433-4268. Pre/Post Natal Relaxation and Massage
Lifeworks (403) 244-4469. Personal Growth and Counselling
Ending the Cycle of Abuse (403) 266-4111 YWCA offers free counselling and workshops for both partners in the relationship
A Woman's Place Book Store (403) 263-5256
Alberta Wholistic Recovery Service (403) 239-7718
Center for Family Well Being (403) 291-0845
Family Chiropractic Center (403) 247-2947
Hands in Motion Pregnancy Massage (403) 247-2947
Joan Cosway-Hayes, Reflexologist (403) 289-9902
Dr. Linda Kodnar, ND Naturopathic Practitioner (403) 278-0867
Over the Edge Apothecary email: (oneman@tic.ab.ca)
Sol-Luna Homeopathy (403) 640-2381
True Essence Aromatherapy (403) 283-8783
Foothills College of Massage (403) 255-4445
Cathy Marricks, Homeopath (403) 640-2381
Dr. Lori Kardal, Pediatrician (403) 252-6651

CRISIS SERVICES (24 HOURS)

Distress Centre Crisis Line (403) 266-1605
Calgary Women's Emergency Shelter (403) 232-8717
Sheriff King Home (403) 266-0707
Parents Anonymous Stress Line (403) 265-1117
Children's Cottage (403) 246-2273
Emergency Social Services (403) 270-5335
Child Abuse Hot Line Dial 0 Ask for Zenith 1234
Telecare Phone Counselling (403) 266-0700
Support Center for Battered Women (403) 266-4111

SPECIAL NEEDS

Calgary Parents of Multiple Births Association (403) 274-8703
Ups and Downs (403) 235-2961
Alexandra Community Health Center (403) 266-2622
Calgary Health Services Best Beginning Program (403) 228-8221
Calgary Immigrant Women's Association (403) 263-4414
Calgary Pregnancy Care Center (403) 269-3110
Calgary Urban Project Society CUPS (403) 221-8780
Louise Dean School for Pregnant & Parenting Teens (403) 777-7630
SIDS Parent Support Group (403) 265-7437
Caring Beyond (24 Hour) 294-1131
Compassionate Friends (403) 259-7914

BIRTH CONTROL AND CONCEPTION

PC-2000 Fertility Tester (403)464-2605 (403)270-0440 1-800-661-4251
Calgary Billings Center (403)541-1091
Planned Parenthood Alberta (403)283-8591
Serena Calgary Natural Family Planning (403)252-9298
Calgary Birth Control Action Line (403)230-4442

PARENTING SITES ON THE INTERNET

Pregnancy Tips – http://calgary.shaw.wave.ca/pregnancytips
Child Friendly Calgary – http://incalgary.com/children.htm
The National Parenting Center – http://www.mpc.com
The Family – http://www.uvol.com/family
Family Web's – http://familyweb.com
Kidsource – http://www.kidsource.com
Between Moms – http://www.cadvision.com/moms
Welcome to the Parent Soup – http://www.parentsoup.com
La Leche League International – http://www.lalecheleague.org
Calgary's Child Magazine – http://www.calgaryschild.com

UNITED STATES

To assemble your health team in the United States contact any of the following assocations for the most current referrals on the best birth physicians, independent midwives, doulas, professional labor support, birth clinics, breastfeeding support and postnatal support to assemble a health team in your city.

BIRTH SERVICES

American Association of Naturopathic Physicians

#322, 2366 Eastlake Avenue, Seattle, WA 98102 (206) 323-7610
American College of Home Obstetrics
P.O. Box 508, Oak Park, IL 60303 (708) 383-1461
American College of Nurse-Midwives
#900, 818 Connecticut Avenue NW, Washington, DC (202) 728-9860
American Osteopathic Board of General Practice
330 E. Algonquin Road, Arlington Heights, IL 60005 (708) 635-8477
Doulas of North America
11000 – 23rd Avenue East, Seattle, WA 98112
Farm Midwifery Center
One of the best places for birth in the United States
48 The Farm, Summertown, TN 38483 (615) 964-2293
Friends of Midwives
PO Box 3188, Boston, MA 02130
Informed Birth and Parenting
PO Box 3675, Ann Arbor, MI 48106 (313) 662-6857
International Childbirth Education Association
P.O. Box 20048, Minneapolis, MN 55420 (612) 854-8660
Midwifery Today
PO Box 2672-MP, Eugene, OR 97402
Midwives Alliance of North America
PO Box 175, Newton, KS 67114 (316) 283-4543
National Association of Childbirth Assistants
205 Copco Lane, San Jose, CA 95123 (408) 225-9167
National Association of Independant Childbearing Centers
3123 Gottschall Road, Perkiomenville, PA 18074 (215) 234-8068
National Association of Parents and Professionals for Safe Alternatives in Childbirth
Route l, Box 646, Marble Hill, MO 63764 (314) 238-2010

MIDWIFERY ORGANIZATIONS
Alabama Midwives Association
1610 Douglas St. SE, Cullman, AL 35055 (205) 734-6123
Midwives Association of Alaska
14870 Snowshoe Lane, AK 99516 (907) 345-1398
Arizona Associations of Midwives
8129 N. 35TH Avenue, Phoenix, AZ 85051 (602) 942-0900
Arkansas Association of Midwives
4322 Country Club Boulevard, Little Rock, AR 72207
California Association of Midwives
PO Box 417854, Sacramento, CA 95841 (800) 829-5791

Colorado Midwives Association
PO Box 1067, Boulder, CO 80306
Connecticut Midwives Alliance
61 High Street, Terryville, CT 06786 (203) 585-1906
Midwives Association of Florida
PO Box 557342, Miami, FL 33255 (813) 274-6404
Georgia Midwifery Association
PO Box 29633, Atlanta, GA 30359 (404) 381-2339
Midwives Alliance of Hawaii
15, 940 Puna Wai Street, Pahoa, HI 96778 (808) 956-8026
Idaho Midwifery Council
2115 N 29th, Boise, ID 83703 (208) 343-8251
Illinois Alliance of Midwives
5703 Hillcrest, Richmond, IL 60071 (815) 678-7531
Indiana Midwives Association
10017 East 1000 S, Upland, IN 46989
Iowa Midwives
RR 1, Box 172A, Mount Sterling, IA 52573 (319) 494-5512
Kansas Midwives Association
8209 SE Lake Road, Whitewater, KS 67154 (316) 799-1044
Kentucky Midwives Alliance
PO Box 856, Paris, KY 40362 (502) 233-9213
Lousiana Midwives Association
PO Box 65154, Baton Rouge, LA 70896-5154
Midwives of Main
PO Box 1, Saint Albans, ME 04971 (207) 938-2094
Chesapeake Midwifery Guild
6740 Cedar Lane, Columbia, MD 21044 (410) 531-5839
Massachusetts Midwives Alliance
PO Box 112, Fiskdale, MA 01518 (508) 376-8201
Michigan Midwives Assocation
4220 Loop Road, Herperia, MI 49421 (616) 861-2234
Minnesota Midwives Guild
PO Box 57, Hendrum, MN 56550 (218) 861-6172
Mississippi Midwives Alliance
Route l, PO Box 135-S, Cleveland, MS 38732
Missouri Midwives Association
PO Box 382, El Dorado Springs, MO 64744 (573) 392-BABY
Montana Midwives Association
200 Woodworth Avenue, Missoula, MT 59801
Nebraska Midwives Association

9508 Burdette, Omaha, NE 68134 (402) 491-3833
Nevada Midwives Association
6695 Eastridge Drive, Reno, NV (702) 367-3323
New Hampshire Midwives Association
20 Coffins Court, Portsmouth, NH 03801 (603) 433-1203
New Jersey Friends of Midwives
70 Mount Vernon Road, Columbia, NJ 07832 (908) 362-6508
New Mexico Midwives Association
PO Box 40647, Albuquerque, NM 87196 (505) 265-2782
Midwives Alliance of New York
PO Box 1000, Warwick, NY 10990 (914) 986-2995
North Carolina Midwives Alliance
PO Box 2156, Rutherfordton, NC 28139 (704) 675-5316
North Dakota Midwives
206 Cheyenne Avenue, Bismarck, ND 58501 (701) 258-5609
Ohio Midwives Alliance
58 South Center Street, West Jefferson, OH 43162 (614) 879-8974
Oklahoma Midwives Alliance
PO Box 54213, Tulsa, OK 74155 (918) 357-3374
Oregon Midwifery Council
5705 NE Duniway, Dayton, OR 97114 (503) 864-2106
Pennsylvania Midwives Association
11267 Mountain Road, Orrstown, PA 17244 (717) 532-9145
Rhode Island Midwives
PO Box 204, Barrington, RI 02806
South Carolina Midwives Association
1644 Charlestown, Leesville, SC 29070 (803) 894-3829
South Dakota Midwives
1017 South Washington Street, Aberdeen, SD 57401 (701) 852-2822
Tennessee Midwives Association
720 Woodmere Drive, Nashville, TN 37217 (615) 367-1119
The Farm Midwives Association
42 Drakes Lane, Summertown, TN 38483
Association of Texas Midwives
603 West 13th Street, Austin, TX 78701 (512) 928-2311
Utah Midwives Association
1160 Sego Lily Drive, Sandy, UT 84094
Vermont Midwives Alliance
30 Park Street, Barre, VT 05641 ((802) 476-7056
Commonwealth Midwives Alliance
Route 2, PO Box 607, Amishville, VA 22022

Midwives Association of Washington State
#300, 2524 16th Avenue, Seattle, WA 98144 (206) 860-4120
Midwives Alliance of West Virginia
NBU #28, Greenwood, WV 26360 (304) 653-4973
Wisconsin Guild of Midwives
East 453 County Road, Scandinavia, WI 54977 (715) 467-2372
Alliance of Wisconsin Midwives
Trout Creek Road, PO Box 210, Soldier Grove, WI 54655
Midwives Alliance of Wyoming
PO Box 5131, Cheyenne, WY 82003

PRENATAL CLASSES
American Society for Lamaze
#300, 1101 Connecticut Avenue NW, Washington, DC 20036 (202) 857-1128
The Bradley Method of Husband-Coached Childbirth
Box 5224, Sherman Oaks, CA 91413-5224 (818) 788-6662 and (1-800) 423-2397
Read Natural Childbirth Foundation Inc.
P.O. Box 150956, San Rafael, CA 94915 (415) 456-8462
NAPSAC National Directory of Prenatal and Alternative Birth Services
Route 1, Box 646, Marble Hill, MO 63764-9725

BREASTFEEDING
La Leche League International
PO Box 1209, 9616 Minneapolis Avenue, Franklin Park, IL 60131-8209 1-800-LA-LECHE, (708) 455-7730. The La Leche League offers optional monthly support meetings and free telephone assistance to breastfeeding moms. La Leche League in your city can also be found by looking in the white pages of your telephone directory. This organization is known throughout the world. You will find it staffed with friendly, knowledgeable mothers who live in your city.

MULTIPLE BIRTHS
Center for Study of Multiple Births #476, 333 Superior Street, Chicago, IL 60611 (312) 266-9093
Twin Services P.O. Box 10066, Berkeley, CA 94709 (415) 524-0863
Triplet Connection P.O. Box 99571, Stockton, CA 95209 (209) 474-0885

CESAREAN PREVENTION

International Cesarean Awareness Movement
1304 Kingsdale Avenue, Redondo Beach, CA 90278 (310) 542-6400
Cesarean Support Education and Concern Inc.
10 Speen Street, Farmingham, MA 01701 (508) 820-2760

BEREAVEMENT

A.M.E.N.D. 4324 Berrywick Terrace, St. Lois, MO 63128
(314) 487-7582
Compassionate Friends P.O. Box 3696, Oak Brook, IL 70622-3696 (708)
990-0010
Unite Inc. 7600 Central Avenue, Philadelphia, PA 19111
(215) 728-2082

INFERTILITY

American Fertility Society #200, 2140 – 11th Ave.S.Birmingham, AL 35205
(205) 933-8494
Barren Foundation #2408, 65 E Wacker Place, Chicago, IL 60601 (312)
782-1356
Center for Surrogate Parenting 8383 Wilshire Blvd. Beverly Hills,CA
90211(213)655-1974
DES Action #510, 1615 Broadway, Oakland, CA 94612 (415) 465-4011
Society of Assisted Reproductive Technology #200, 2140 – 11th Avenue S.
Birmingham, AL 35205-2800 (205) 933-8494
Surrogates by Choice P.O. Box 05257, Detroit, MI 48205 (313) 839-4946

POSTNATAL SUPPORT

Formerly Employed Mothers at the Leading Edge
PO Box 31, Elmhurst, IL 60126 (708) 941-3553
A support and advocacy group for women taking time out from paid
employment to raise their children at home. More than seventy chapters
across the United States with activities including regular meetings,
playgroups, baby-sitting co-ops, membership directory, Mom's Night Out
activities and a support system in times of personal need.

Mothers at Home
8210A Old Courthouse Road, Vienna, VA 22182 (703) 827-5903
Supports moms who choose to stay at home to raise their families.
Publishes a monthly journal that serves as a networking mechanism for
mothers all over the United States. It includes poetry, research articles,
health and safety issues, artwork, and more, all contributed by mothers.

Warriors

4504 N 47, Milwaukee, WI 53218 (414) 444-0220
Offers new mothers peer counseling and emotional support. They have a Mom's Helpline to teach self-advocacy and to counsel and validate women in their choices or lack of choices.

Match

PO Box 123, Annandale, VA 22003 (703) 791-6264
Provides networking, advocacy and support for women who have chosen to combine motherhood and a career based from home.

The Compleat Mother

RR #3, Clifford, Ontario, Canada NOG lMO (519) 327-8785
An informal, world-wide support network for mothers. Publishes a quarterly magazine covering the newest discoveries in the field of pregnancy, childbirth and breastfeeding as well as including an informal chat section where real mothers voice their philosophy, ideas, and discoveries on motherhood.

MAGAZINES

The Mother Is Me

PO Box 5174, Dover, NH, 03821 (603) 743-6828
An alternative publication on the motherhood experience.

The Doula – Mothering the Mother

PO Box 71, Santa Cruz, CA 95063-0071
Birth and breastfeeding stories, insights, parenting and home schooling.

Birth Gazette

42-C The Farm, Sumertown, TN 38483 (615) 964-3798
State of the art quarterly magazine covering the practice, the politics, techniques, economics, folklore and the emotion of childbirth and reproduction.

Mother Tongue

PO Box 3061, Asherville, NC 28802 (704) 665-4572
A progressive parenting source of items, ideas and interests.

Mothering Magazine

PO Box 1690, Sante Fe, NM 87504
The most comprehensive and accurate coverage of childbirth today.

1

First Month

Take your home pregnancy test with your partner. Let him share in the excitement or surprise. London Drug stores sell their pregnancy test for less than ten dollars. Most pregnancy tests can be used as early as three weeks after the first day of your last period.

When do you tell people that you are pregnant? Tell your family first! Your family will not want to hear about such an important event from other people – news does travel fast! Your friends should be the next to know and then the people that you work with. Be careful at work . . . your boss may not want to find out from the person at the front desk. Tell all of the other interested parties when you feel comfortable. For some, this is immediately and for others it may be three or four months down the road.

Mothers and mothers-in-law are notorious for scheduling their flights a week before the baby's due date and then asking you every day when you plan to have the baby, especially if this is a first grandchild. Each day you give your baby in your womb is a precious gift only you can give. Your first baby may easily want to stay in your womb for two or three weeks after your estimated due date of forty weeks, growing and developing safely even throughout the last stages of your labor and delivery when your baby's lungs mature by a hormone released by your body during labor.

Being pregnant isn't like anything you have ever experienced. Get ready to accept that many things will change: the way you feel, the way you look, the way some people talk to you and treat you. You will be changing some of your own ideas as well about parenting once you become a parent. Your sleep habits will change, your eating habits will change to support the growth of your baby, you may experience highs and lows in your energy and emotions, and for some women even their dreams change. Each pregnancy, every woman and every baby is very different from the next. You will also find that each stage of your pregnancy is different from the next, giving you new challenges and joy as your baby grows and takes form within you.

Hormones altered by pregnancy can loosen up joints, especially your hips. Find a chiropractor who has experience working with pregnant women if you are experiencing back pain during any stage of your pregnancy. Wearable magnets from Nikken or BMI can ease many types of back pain during pregnancy, and the magnets can be shifted to your abdominal area to reduce nausea.

Calculating Your Due Date

To calculate the estimated arrival of your baby take the first day of your last period and count forward 42 weeks and mark it on your calendar.

Counting fourteen days after the first day of your last period will give you the date of conception if your cycle is usually 28 days long.

Henci Goer, childbirth researcher and author of *Obstetric Myths Versus Research Realities*, 1995, has reported studies that show the median gestational length exceeds 280 days among healthy, white, middle-class women. Babies of first-time mothers have an average gestational length of 38 to 42 weeks and longer. No person and no machine can give you the exact date your baby will be ready to be born. Sheila Kitzinger, world-renown childbirth educator and researcher, reports that seven out of ten babies arrive 10 days after a due date of forty weeks. The most exact figure would then be forty-two weeks from the first day of your last period less three days.

Prenatal Vitamins

The day you become aware that you are pregnant, go to a health food store and purchase prenatal vitamins. Health food stores offer the best value for your money on prenatal vitamins and are usually made allergy-free, providing an extra benefit for you and your baby. Plan to take one-a-day throughout each stage of your pregnancy and for the first six months after the birth of your baby. Pregnancy places a high demand on your physical and emotional body, and by giving yourself extra nutritional support at this time you and your baby will benefit greatly. Taking liquid organic colloidal minerals can also give your body and baby the extra nutritional support that is not always available in the foods we eat.

Preventing Birth Defects

The March of Dimes has conclusive research that many birth defects can be prevented by taking folic acid (a B vitamin) supplement, especially for the month before you are pregnant and for the first three months of pregnancy. They suggest you consume 0.4 milligrams of folic acid every day. Folic acid is found mainly in green leafy vegetables, beans, asparagus, citrus fruits and juices, whole grain foods and liver. It is difficult to get enough folic acid through diet alone, so it is important to make up the difference by taking a prenatal vitamin supplement. Zinc is also an important mineral that can prevent birth defects.

The latest research from Nobel Peace Prize Nominee Dr. Joel Wallich, BS, DVM, ND, shows that pregnant women from around the world who naturally consume extra minerals during pregnancy have fewer or no birth defects.

Natural Remedies for Morning Sickness

Do soda crackers really work? Yes! Leave a package on your bedside table and eat a few before you get up in the morning. Keep some small packages of crackers in your purse in case nausea strikes while you are away from the house.

- Chew on licorice-tasting fennel seeds to calm queasiness.
- Fresh grated ginger and fennel seeds make a comforting tea to settle your stomach. Ginger can be purchased at your grocery store in the fresh vegetable section.
- Try eating your favorite foods from childhood, like ginger ale, jello or whatever your mother fed you when you weren't feeling well.
- Always get up slowly in the morning and take small breaks throughout the day with your feet elevated.
- Hot teas may help, especially spearmint or peppermint, known to be good for indigestion, or try the excellent "women's tea" known as red raspberry-leaf tea. If cold is more appealing, make popsicles or ice chips with the teas.
- Take short walks in the fresh air whenever possible.
- Drink bottled or purified water to flush your system.
- If you feel as though your stomach is not digesting food well, increase your consumption of raw, enzyme-rich foods. Fresh canteloupe, papaya and pineapple have the highest naturally occurring enzymes of all foods and help a great deal with digestion.
- Make sure you are napping at least once a day to allow your body to recharge. Even a short nap can help you to feel stronger.
- Some health professionals are recommending one tablet of Vitamin B6, in the amount of 50 mg to 100 mg before bed, and this has worked extremely well for some women. Single B vitamins should be used only for short periods of time. Switch to a B-complex vitamin after a two-week period.
- There is a strong connection between nausea during pregnancy and low blood-sugar levels. Make sure you are eating small meals throughout the day to keep your blood-sugar level up throughout the day and evening.
- A high protein snack before bed can help to alleviate some symptoms.
- Try powdered ginger root in capsules, three capsules a day.
- Slippery elm is a soothing and strengthening herb for the stomach. It has as much nutrition as oatmeal and is so gentle that it can be retained by the most sensitive stomach. It can be taken in powdered form in capsules or made into a gruel.
- Carry raisins, raw almonds, rice cakes or whole-wheat crackers with you so

that you can keep your blood-sugar level up.

- Blue green algae, such as spirulina, is very high in protein and very easy to digest. Spirulina powder can be mixed with mashed bananas or other fruit and provides excellent nutritional support. It can be taken in tablet form as well.
- Try increasing your water intake to six glasses a day.
- Many women find sea-bands useful. These are elastic bracelets with a plastic button that are worn on the wrist to put compression on an acupressure point that controls nausea. These can be worn 24 hours a day.
- According to the newest research, morning sickness may be a healthy and protective way for a woman's body to reject foods that may be harmful to her baby. There is less incidence of miscarriage in women who experience morning sickness. Unless vomiting is making a woman dehydrated, she should be reassured that her baby is very healthy and vomiting will subside at the end of the first trimester when the baby's development is less sensitive to toxins.
- Never take any prescription or non-prescription drugs for your nausea. Benedictin, in the past prescribed by some doctors for the nausea of pregnancy has been associated with birth defects such as cleft palate and heart deformities.
- Consult a midwife or homeopath if you find your morning sickness is not alleviated by the above remedies. Reasons for nausea can be many and varied and getting at the cause can give better direction to the remedy.

Choosing Your Health Team

Create your health team now. The more responsibility you take for your pregnancy and childbirth, the better the results will be. Be an active participant in your prenatal care. Use your health team as a resource; not an authority. One of the reasons there are so many medical interventions in hospitals, which lead to complications, is because women have not been taught to trust in their ability to deliver naturally and without fear. The full responsibility for the health of the mother and the baby is then shifted unfairly to the doctor's and the nurse's shoulders.

Visit the free-standing birthing center in your city and find out what they have to offer you. Free-standing means to stand free from hospital rules and regulations. Many of the free-standing birthing centers offer you unlimited options for your birth, including water births. Some general practitioners are delivering babies again. You may want to use your family doctor along with a doula who will stay with you throughout your entire labor and delivery. You may decide to have a home birth, assisted by a midwife support team during your pregnancy, labor, delivery and at home with your baby. Midwives will often work on a sliding fee to accommodate mothers of all incomes, which can be an added bonus. In many countries of the world, including Great Britain, midwives are publicly funded so that every woman can have a choice for the birth of her baby.

After researching your options, it will soon become clear which method of childbirth you will be most comfortable with. To create your health team you may want to include all or some of the following:

1. Midwife, General Practitioner, Obstetrician, Osteopath, or Naturopath
2. Labor Support Coach – Midwife, Doula or Professional Labor Support
3. Birth Partner – Your Partner or Female Relative or Friend
4. Childbirth Educator – For Prenatal Classes
5. Breastfeeding Support – Neighborhood La Leche Group or Breastfeeding Clinic
6. Postnatal Care – Midwife or Doula

Your nearest Childbirth Association or Midwives Association can be an excellent resource center for finding out what your city has to offer. Visit your nearest office for a cup of tea and free information on what your area has to offer. The Childbirth Resource Directory in this guidebook will refer you to the many services that are offered to new mothers in the areas of pregnancy, childbirth, breastfeeding and newborn care. By taking advantage of these services you will create an excellent support team in your city or town for yourself and your baby.

When interviewing health team members, book your appointment for a consultation only. Remind the receptionist upon your arrival that you wish to meet with the doctor in his office for a consultation. If you have chosen your family general practitioner to continue caring for you throughout your pregnancy, make sure that they will be attending the birth of your baby as well. Continuity of care is important for all members on your health team.

Follow your intuition and your feelings when choosing your health team. You have a vision of how you wish your labor and delivery to be; if you find it difficult to get agreement on your birth plan, switch to another caregiver. Make sure your health professionals make time to answer all your questions and that you feel confident in their approach. Don't be surprised if you have to fire your doctor or if he fires you. A good working relationship is important for both of you. What is most important is that you both have the same philosophies about birth.

Take your time at the beginning of your pregnancy to create a health team that you will be completely at ease with. Your vision of your birth is as unique as you are, and you deserve to have support for it. When choosing your health team, follow your intuition, and ask yourself the following questions:

1. Does my doctor or midwife listen to me?

2. Does my doctor or midwife directly answer all of my questions?
3. Do I feel comfortable with my doctor or midwife?
4. Do I feel respected by my doctor or midwife?
5. Do I trust my doctor or midwife?

The most empowering part of pregnancy and childbirth is the role you play. By creating a health team and place of birth most comfortable for you, you will become more confident and positive about your role ahead.

When you are discussing birth issues with your doctor or midwife, ask under what circumstances would they perform an episiotomy, induction or cesarean. Ask how their rates of intervention compare to other health professionals in your city or town. Ask if they have experience with normal birth and what percentage of women experience normal birth with them. Find out if you will have professional labor support available to you throughout the entire labor or if the physician only attends during the last few moments of delivery. Don't be surprised that you may be left alone for long periods of time if you are having your baby in a hospital. It is critical to plan for professional labor support to be with you at all times if this will be your first baby.

Be prepared by creating a birth plan to go over with your doctor or midwife. A sample birth plan is shown in the next section and can be modified to fit your design. The following sections explain some of the common medical interventions that can put both you and your baby at risk. Bring this book with you to your first consultation with your health team members and talk about these important issues with your team. It is important to have all members of your health team sign your birth plan and that a copy of your birth plan is kept in your file.

Designing an Easier Labor and a Faster Delivery

If you want an easier labor and a faster delivery with the fewest complications choose a team of midwives. They gently care for you during your prenatal visits, calming fears and gently encouraging you along the way. The purpose of a midwife is to facilitate your labor and delivery. A midwife becomes your experienced coach during labor and delivery, staying with you minute after minute, hour after hour, never leaving your sight until you have reached your goal. Many hospitals are short-staffed and do not have one staff member available to be with you. Your nurse will be dealing with shift changes, the unpredictability of when babies are born, staff shortages and emergencies.

A midwife expects each labor and delivery to be different from the next and is experienced at watching and waiting. A midwife has the patience to stay with you during a prolonged labor and has tools to deal with almost any contingency that may arise. A midwife provides excellent aftercare, as she will see you and your baby in your home for the first few days after your birth. A mother also needs nurturing at this time, and you will find your concerns and questions easily answered by telephone, whether your concern is for yourself or for your new baby. A midwife will see that your baby has a calm and gentle entry into this world. If you are choosing to give birth in a hospital you can bring a midwife, doula or professional labor assistant in with you if you choose.

What You Need to Know Before You Have Your Baby: Choosing a Good Birth Practitioner

Excerpted from, Take This Book to the Obstetrician with You, *Karla Morales and Charles B. Inlander 1991*

The commonly held wisdom in the field of obstetrics is that 90% of all pregnant women are capable of delivering normally without any help or interference. Some experts say this is a conservative figure and that somewhere between 93% and 96% of women experiencing normal births is more realistic. Even with the medical intervention that occurs in the majority of births in this country, most women go through pregnancy and delivery with few or no complications.

However, doctors do make mistakes. Improper birth-related treatment has consistently placed high on the list of the top ten malpractice claims compiled annually by St. Paul Fire and Marine Insurance Company, the largest private malpractice insurer in the country. In 1988, improper birth-related treatment was the second most frequent malpractice allegation. The company tallies the average cost for birth-related malpractice claims at $129,123.

Doctor-shopping would be a whole lot easier if someone would profile the malpracticing obstetrician; that is, inventory the typical traits of obstetricians who incur high malpractice risk, either for what they do or for what they do not do. Well, someone has; and who better to have done so than a lawyer for the defense, who along with the doctor and the consumer is the other person most privy to the practices and actions that result in a charge of malpractice.

"Dunn's Rule" is what Lee J. Dunn, Jr, J.D., a partner in the Boston Firm of Dunn and Auton, calls this profile, based on his nearly twenty years of experience in medical malpractice suits, plus conversations with many other defense lawyers and plaintiffs' attorneys. "Time after time experience has shown me and many others that the rule holds true." Apparently consumers are not the only ones hungry for such an analysis. We caught up with Dunn not long after a presentation he made at an update on medicolegal issues in obstetrics and gynecology, presented by the Harvard Medical School.

According to Dunn, cases with significant verdicts or settlements tend to fall into at least one and usually two or more of the following categories:

1. The physician is a graduate of a foreign medical school or, if trained in the U.S. is over 50 years of age and not board-certified: with foreign medical

school graduates, Dunn says, the problem is not necessarily one of a poorer medical education, but more a matter of inability to communicate effectively in colloquial English. The issue of age and board-certification status, in his view, to often comes down to a lag in knowledge and skills – the newest practices and latest changes in obstetrics, which is probably the fastest changing area of medicine.

2. The cases occur in a community hospital does not have the advantages of a tertiary care hospital with its medical residents (one more guardian at the gate), house officers, stringent peer review system, and other steps to help ensure quality, according to Dunn.

3. Abuse of oxytocin, administered to induce or hasten labor, when administered for other than sound clinical reasons. This practice, Dunn explains, can become more a matter of convenience for the physician than a medical necessity.

4. Poor medical record-keeping reflecting an overall sloppiness.

5. The physician delivers more than 300 babies a year. Two problems derive from this, the latest addition to Dunn's Rule: the practitioner is just too busy to give proper care and too often delegates care to nurses or others who are not prepared for emergencies or complications that may arise.

While most pregnancies do not run a high risk of complication or carry a risk of negligent or improper care, your doctor's competence will have great impact on your chances of being malpracticed on. The fact is, most consumers spend more time selecting their roofer than they do choosing someone to provide their medical care. The earlier you start to shop for the right birth practitioner, the better. This way you have the time to approach the process from a consumerist perspective – ask the right questions, evaluate the answers, and choose among your various options. And an early start gives you enough leeway to change practitioners, if you desire, before the final stage of the journey: labor and delivery.

Choosing a birth practitioner isn't easy. It is a process filled with questions, both for the prospective provider and for yourself, but the right choice can save you heartbreak and money. After all, bad medical care costs much more than good medical care: it takes its toll on your health and your family, as well as on your pocketbook.

2

Second Month

"Childbirth is a major milestone in a woman's life. It can be a pivotal, positive and empowering experience for a woman." states Dr. Carolyn DeMarco. By taking charge of your pregnancy and the birth of your baby you will enjoy the journey as well as the destination.

Now is the time to read as much as you can, talk to professionals and mothers about birth and to work on creating your birth plan and health team for a normal, active birth for you and your baby.

Your Prenatal Visits

Be informed and get information from your health team at every checkup. Throughout the month, write out a list of questions and keep them in your purse; this will save you from "I forgot to ask about...." Ask your questions when you are being examined. No question is too trivial for your peace of mind. Your prenatal check-ups will usually include blood-pressure checks, urine checks and weight checks. When you have many questions, ask the receptionist to book in extra time for you.

Stay in control throughout the entire process. Learn to listen to your body. Inform yourself, read, talk and don't be shy about the physical details. You can lead your health team by being adamant or firm about what you want to take place. Don't settle for less than comfort with your health care team. Trust your feelings about what you want. Being pregnant and birthing your baby doesn't happen every day. If your intuition or instincts are telling you that something is wrong, follow up on that by talking to someone on your team.

One emotion most mothers face is fear. Another one is worry. Deal with both of these emotions as they come up. By asking questions you will eliminate most of your fear and worry. A quick phone call or visit allows most matters to be easily resolved, and your peace of mind during this time is worth it. Bring your Birth Plan along with you at every visit. If you run out of questions you can refer to your plan and talk about each aspect of it in detail.

Birth Plan

Create your birth plan now. Choreograph your baby's first day. Plan every detail of what will be the most exciting and remembered time of your life. As in life, you are the director, script writer, prop person and star. You choose who you wish to have around you in your production. Discuss with your partner and your health team what you want to happen at your labor and delivery. Communicate your wishes by having them prepared in advance. The more you know and are prepared for in advance, the less stress you deal with when you are doing your work during labor.

PERSONAL BIRTH PLAN

Birth Plan of: _____ mother and _____ father.
Thank you for choosing to be a part of our health team. We are expecting the arrival of our new baby on or about _____.

It is our belief that birth is a natural event in the reproductive life of a woman. If a medical problem should arise we expect both the problem and the risks and benefits of any proposed procedure, as well as any natural alternatives to be discussed with us. We would like time alone to consider our options.

We have educated ourselves through monthly prenatal medical appointments, taking prenatal classes and reading current medical research on pregnancy and childbirth. It is very important that we have an unmedicated birth. We appreciate your assistance in guiding us safely through the birth process and your support for the following preferences:

YES	NO	
❐	❐	Inductions to force or speed up labor.
❐	❐	I.V.s
❐	❐	Epidural or Spinal Block.
❐	❐	Catheters.
❐	❐	Continual Mechanical Fetal Monitoring.
❐	❐	Ultrasound.
❐	❐	Episiotomy.
❐	❐	Breaking of waters or stripping of membranes.
❐	❐	Unnecessary vaginal exams.
❐	❐	Time limit on labor or delivery.

YES	NO	
❑	❑	Midwife or doula present at labor and delivery.
❑	❑	Walking and changing position as much as possible.
❑	❑	Baby monitored manually.
❑	❑	Squatting bar on the birthing bed for the delivery.
❑	❑	Shower and bath tub available.
❑	❑	Mirror available for the final stage of labor and delivery.
❑	❑	Sex of baby discovered naturally.
❑	❑	Baby placed upon mother immediately after birth to help modulate baby's temperature and breathing.
❑	❑	Breastfeed baby within the first few minutes of birth.
❑	❑	Umbilical cord left on as long as it continues to pulse.
❑	❑	Partner to cut the umbilical cord.
❑	❑	Baby to be in the room with mother at all times.
❑	❑	Should a cesarean section become necessary partner and professional labor assistant to attend mother at all times.
❑	❑	Local rather than a general anesthetic if a cesarean is necessary.
❑	❑	Mother is to be able to welcome baby gently with dim lights, a warm room, baby placed immediately upon mother's breast, warm blankets to be placed over baby and time given for mother and baby to relax and attach.
❑	❑	To labor and give birth in the same place.
❑	❑	Mother is to be able to do what she chooses.
❑	❑	To eat and drink as wanted.
❑	❑	To have minimum interference.
❑	❑	To be in quiet, peaceful surroundings.
❑	❑	To maintain a spiritual perspective throughout the birth.

YES	NO	
☐	☐	To have other children present.
☐	☐	To have other supportive people present.
☐	☐	To be in a birthing center.
☐	☐	To have access to a birthing room and a midwife in a hospital.
☐	☐	To give birth at home with professionals experienced in normal childbirth.
☐	☐	To have a safe, normal, joyful birth.

_____ Signature of Mother _____ Date

Wainer Cohen and Estner state, "Occasionally, once in a while, infrequently, not routinely, each medical or obstetrical procedure has a place at birth. For the most part, however, it is best to depend on trusted, knowledgeable individuals rather than technology at birth. A human ear to check the fetal heart. Human hands and minds to assess health, in conjunction with feelings and sensory judgment reported by each mother. Birth is a state of wellness. When normal, healthy women say no to the purveyors of technology, the believers in machines, they say a confident and loving yes to themselves and their babies. One physician remarks, 'Everyone has their favorite interventions. Dr. A. insists upon IVs but could care less about monitors. Dr. B. demands the use of monitors, but has a nonchalant attitude about IVs.' Perhaps the dissension within the field will ultimately provide women with the fuel they need to refuse all but the most necessary interventions."

Your Emotional Health

Your baby experiences the wide range of emotions you feel. Find a way now to deal with the negative emotions and stress that accumulate daily. What relaxes you? A warm bath, a walk in the fresh air, reading, sewing, hobbies or crafts or exercise can all help you to release your emotions by relaxing you. Incorporate your favorite de-stressing activity into every day so that you can release stress as it comes up.

Amniocentesis

An amniocentesis test can be done to determine whether your baby has certain genetic defects. Usually your health plan will cover the cost of the test if you will deliver your baby after your 35th birthday. The risks to you and your baby from this test include infection, hemorrhage, fetal damage, miscarriage, embolism, premature labor, damage to uterine and placental vessels, puncture of the umbilical cord causing cerebral damage, sudden deaths and unexplained respiratory problems for babies at birth. This test has not proven to be accurate on either positive or negative results. The test may show something as wrong when everything is fine. It can easily miss a problem should one exist.

An amniocentesis test is never mandatory. Make sure both you and your partner are made aware of the risks involved. The procedure will be done only after the ultrasound shows that you are at a later stage of pregnancy. During the procedure you lie on your back with your head slightly elevated to relax the abdominal muscles. Your lower abdomen is cleansed with an antiseptic solution and covered with sterile drapes. A needle is then inserted through the skin and into the uterus. Amniotic fluid is withdrawn into the syringe for laboratory testing. Results take at least six weeks, bringing you well into your second trimester before you are informed of them.

If you arrange for an amniocentesis test you must also schedule two days of rest in bed immediately after the test. Your body will need to repair the needle puncture to your womb and to replace the amniotic fluid. Do not exert yourself, avoid any heavy lifting and do not have sexual intercourse the first 24 hours following your test. If you experience any of the following after the first 48 hours following the test, contact your health team immediately: leaking of fluid from the vagina, abdominal pain, cramping or fever.

The scientific validity of amniocentesis has yet to be proven. The inherent health risks have. Make sure you read all the studies before you choose this test. Many hospitals are now including a short seminar on some of the risks and side effects of this procedure. Ask your health team about the accuracy level of this test before you undertake it and have them explain the rate of error as well. The best way to make certain your baby is healthy is to eat well and rest well. Your health is of the utmost importance to the health of your baby. Taking the best care of yourself and your baby now can give you the best assurance of good health for all.

Chorionic Villus Sampling – The New Amniocentesis

Newsweek Magazine in 1992 reported that two separate studies have established a link between the use of chorionic villus sampling (CVS) and birth defects. The Oxford study and the Humana-Michael Reese Hospital in Chicago both found limb abnormalities in babies who had CVS in utero. The affected children in these studies were born with missing or shortened fingers and toes.

Chorionic villus sampling, which was introduced to the United States in the mid-1980s, consists of removing a small piece of tissue from the chorionic villi, the hairlike projections on the outermost layer of the amniotic sac. Fetal cells present in this tissue are then analyzed and screened for genetic anomalies.

Several hospitals have ceased to perform CVS and the National Institute of Health will soon recommend that all women be informed of the risk before agreeing to this procedure.

The Birth Gazette (Summer 1992) reports that when an expensive test which is undergone to assure parents that their children are free of genetic abnormalities leaves these same children disfigured and handicapped, it is time to seriously consider the absurdity of routine technological intervention.

Midwives

Midwives are primary caregivers, meaning they care for pregnant women on their own responsibility like a physician or obstetrician. There are many excellent reasons to have a midwife in attendance throughout your pregnancy, labor and delivery and in your first days home with your new baby. The ideal choice for assistance with the birth of your baby may be a midwife. A midwife promotes low-tech, woman-centered and family-centered approaches to childbirth. Midwives have experienced the process of birth from both sides and have great empathy with the journey you have undertaken. You can count on your midwife to help you understand the birth process from a woman's point of view.

A midwife will become your advocate and coach during your labor and delivery, with yourself, your partner and your health team. A midwife can enable you to have a better birth by giving you the wealth of experience she has accumulated through her own personal experience and through the experience of hundreds of normal, natural births she has assisted. A midwife will provide the nurturing all mothers need throughout their pregnancy. Midwives work in teams so that you do not have to delay or speed up your delivery at the convenience of your health specialist. You will have one midwife to care for you and one midwife to care for your baby. Midwives are prepared to handle almost every emergency and can arrange transport and attend you in the hospital should it become necessary. A midwife will help you to create the calm, loving, supportive environment that all mothers want their babies to have.

A nurse-midwife, working in conjunction with obstetricians in a hospital setting does not have the same authority as an independent midwife or a midwife associated with a free-standing birth clinic. The author of this book was surprised to find out that her nurse-midwives who worked in a hospital actually lost control of her case exactly one week after the expected due date. This in turn led to an induction by the obstetrician in charge of the program. Had she known in advance of this policy and the time limit arbitrarily imposed by the obstetrician on the birth of her first child, she would have used an alternate service and had her baby at nature's convenience.

To locate a midwife with a good reputation contact your midwives association or your local childbirth association located in the Childbirth

Resource Directory. Go to your library and look for books and articles on midwives, talk to friends and relatives for referrals, look in the Yellow Pages under Health Consultants, Birthing Centers, or Midwives and meet and go through your birth plan with them. When you find your midwife, ask for referrals and call to hear how the births went.

Many women are now choosing to have their second baby in the privacy of their own home, having labor support come in to assist during the later stages of labor. If you feel that your home will provide a safer environment for you and your baby or that you may not have your birth plan complied with in your city's hospital, take the time now to read everything you can about home birth or birth in a free-standing birth clinic and find out why women are choosing this option. Whether you plan to have your baby at a hospital, a free-standing birth clinic or at home, a midwife can guide you to a safe birth for you and your baby.

Doulas

A doula provides emotional and physical support during pregnancy, labor, birth and postpartum. Doulas are called childbirth assistants, labor support professionals, birth assistants or birth companions. A doula is hired by you and sometimes provided by the hospital as your professional labor coach. In the best situation you would use an independent doula who you had met and spent time with prior to going into the hospital.

A doula provides explanations of medical procedures, emotional support, advice during pregnancy, and provides exercises and suggestions to make pregnancy more comfortable. She helps with preparation of your birth plan, provides massage and other non-pharmacological pain relief measures, gives positioning suggestions during labor and birth, and provides support for partners. She will also help you to avoid unnecessary medical interventions, assist you with breastfeeding and begin a written record of the birth, along with other possibilities that vary from doula to doula.

In *Mothering the Mother: How a Doula Can Help You Have a Shorter, Easier and Healthier Birth* by Klaus, Kennell and Klaus, 1993, the authors report that, "The presence of a doula:
- Reduces the overall cesarean rate by 50%
- Reduces length of labor by 25%
- Reduces oxytocin (pitocin) use by 40%
- Reduces pain medication by 30%
- Reduces the need for forceps by 40%
- Reduces requests for epidurals by 60%."

A doula will charge anywhere from $200 to $500 for her services depending upon experience and services offered. Some hospitals are now including doula service at no extra charge. To find a doula with the experience you require, call your local association for doulas or midwives in the Childbirth Resource Directory. They will be able to connect you with a doula who matches your birth plan and your personality.

Changing the Birth System

It is up to women as tax payers and consumers to ask our governments, hospitals, doctors and private health plans to provide the services of midwives, doulas and birthing assistants before, during and after birth. If your health plan does not cover it, take the money out of your savings to pay for the extra service of professional labor support.

Many women are tired of the black Model-T Ford Birth Plan that has been offered by the standard obstetric/hospital system for years, and are demanding a custom Red Convertible Birth Plan. Be prepared that you may have to go to another dealership to get another car. Driving off in that red convertible may be the happiest and most empowering day of your life. It is only through knowledge of our options that we will be able to make positive changes in the present birthing system. You can support the various associations now forming to help all women become aware of and have access to safe alternatives in childbirth.

Shopping Tips

Specialty Maternity Clothing stores such as Shirley K Maternity and Thyme Maternity have excellent selections of work and casual clothing, evening wear, lingerie and almost every accessory you may need for your pregnancy. Both Shirley K Maternity and Thyme Maternity stores offer women adjustable clothing so that the pants and skirts purchased will fit you comfortably throughout each stage of your pregnancy. The sales clerks are very supportive and knowledgeable. Go during the early stages of your pregnancy so that you can begin planning your new wardrobe around your first basic purchases.

Plan your first maternity purchase to include a pair of solid colored pants and skirt. You will be able to use your regular blouses for some time so invest your money where you will get the most comfort. Do not let any of your clothing bind you about the waist, hips or breast areas. Your body is growing and changing to accommodate your new baby, and your baby needs room to grow and will appreciate the extra breathing space too.

Comfortable shoes are important. As you gain weight, your feet take the pressure. To avoid ending up with pressure sores on your toes, invest in a couple of pairs of comfortable shoes as the key to your comfort in the early months of your pregnancy.

Purchase a few sets of stretchy leggings in a larger size. They're comfortable, easy to launder and inexpensive. You can mix and match many articles in your existing wardrobe with them. Cockleshells offers excellent pregnancy tights that hold under your waist and will not bind or pull.

What You Need to Know before You Have Your Baby: What You Can Do To Prevent Premature Birth

Excerpted from, Every Pregnant Woman's Guide to Preventing Premature Birth – Reducing the Sixty Proven Risks That Can Lead to Prematurity, *Barbara Luke, ScD. MPH, RN, RD 1995. Barbara Luke is an Associate Professor and Chief, Division of Health Services Research at the University of Michigan Medical School, Department of Obstetrics and Gynecology in Ann Arbor, Michigan. Email address: bluke@umich.edu.*

Prematurity, birth before 37 completed weeks' gestation, is one of the greatest public health problems in the United States today. Each year in the United States there are over four million births. More than one out of ten of these births is premature, or about half a million annually. Half of all deaths to children before their first birthday are due to pregnancy-related factors; nine out of ten of these deaths are due to prematurity and its complications.

Premature babies – preemies – are more than merely small. They are developmentally unprepared for life outside the uterus. If they survive, they are more likely to have problems with growth and development, which can result in physical and mental disabilities. For example, children who were born premature are more likely to have respiratory problems during childhood, as well as a higher incidence of learning disabilities and problems with speech, hearing, and vision. The more premature the infant, the greater the risk of physical and developmental problems during childhood.

Maturity is not the only factor influencing how healthy your baby will be at birth and during infancy: birth weight is also very important. Babies who were "small for gestational age" or "intrauterine growth retarded" have not grown as well as they should have before birth. Many of the same factors cause both prematurity and poor growth before birth. When an infant is both premature and growth-retarded, the risks of death or subsequent disability are greatly increased. Every week prematurity is prevented buys valuable time for your baby to grow and mature, and increases the possibilities that he or she will be healthy and well developed at birth.

Special precautions must be taken for premature babies, including administering oxygen, placing them in heated incubators, feeding them special dietary formulas, muffling extraneous sound and light, and protecting their fragile skin. During recent years, there have been great advances in the care of these infants and improvements in their survival rates, but despite modern technology, there is no substitute for full-term gestation.

Prematurity is a complex, universal problem, with no single cause and no single solution. One of the strongest risk factors is if you have had a prior premature birth. Every woman brings a unique set of factors to each pregnancy. Some risks cannot be changed, such as your genetic background, obstetrical history, and age. Others, such as how much and how often you lift, carry, stand, or make other physical efforts can be changed. Most of the pregnancy books on the market focus on preparing you for labor–an event that lasts thirteen hours on average. My focus is on the whole nine months of your pregnancy: a short-term investment for the lifelong health of your child and the outcome of future pregnancies as well.

While no one can guarantee that your pregnancy will not be premature, by taking the best possible care of yourself and reducing whatever risks you can, you will greatly improve your chances of having a healthy, well-grown baby born at term.

Ask your health team to review with you how to recognize uterine contractions and what to do if and when they occur. Uterine contractions may be perceived as a heaviness in the abdomen or as pain in the middle to lower back, accompanied by a tightening of the uterus. When you feel this heaviness or pain, you should place your hands on your abdomen, at the top of the uterus, to determine if these sensations are accompanied by a tightening or hardening of the uterus. When you squeeze your biceps to make a muscle in your arm, you can feel the muscle go from elastic to hard. When your uterus contracts, you can feel the tightening the same way.

Braxton-Hicks contractions begin during your last trimester and generally increase with intensity as you progress toward your time of birth. You will feel these contractions for very short time periods and then nothing at all for hours or days. These contractions are normal and are your body's way to condition your uterus for delivery.

After you detect uterine contractions, you should determine what you were doing when they occurred. The activities that cause uterine contractions very greatly from woman to woman. For example, for one woman it may be standing on the train during her commute home, carrying groceries, or hanging wallpaper. For another woman, it may be standing for long periods while shopping, carrying a child in her arms, or vacuuming. For a third, it may be an argument with a co-worker or a stressful session of bill paying. Regardless of the activity, it is important for you to:

1. Recognize that uterine contractions are occurring.
2. Identify what activities bring on the contractions.
3. Stop that activity and sit down, or preferably lie down on your left side, until the contractions subside.
4. Drink at least a glass or two of water, since dehydration can also cause uterine contractions.
5. Call your health team immediately and report your contractions.

True labor pains are rhythmic, even during early labor, occurring every fifteen to twenty minutes. After a few hours, the pains occur about every five minutes. False labor occurs when the painful contractions diminish in intensity after a few hours, and labor does not progress. If you experience a sudden gush of fluid from your vagina, with or without painful contractions, call your health team immediately. Since premature contractions are very difficult to stop once they've started, the best way to prevent prematurity is to prevent premature contractions. It is important for you to understand the physical basis of the relationship between standing, stress, and other factors and premature contractions as well.

When you get home, take another close look at the things you take for granted: how much you stand, how often you go up and down stairs – and make changes wherever you can. Walk through your house and evaluate how you can become more organized. Take steps to reduce clutter in your home which in turn will reduce the amount of housework (and physical effort) in your daily life.

Make an effort to decrease the amount of stair climbing, lifting, carrying, standing, and driving you do. Place stools around your kitchen so that it is easier to sit when you are on the telephone or preparing a meal. Turn over the vacuuming to someone else. Lower the volume of the TV and stereo, and cut down on your exposure to noise in other ways if you can. If possible, get help from friends and relatives with food shopping, chores, baby-sitting, and carpooling. When you are with your children spend as much time as you can with them on the floor so that you are not doing so much lifting. Do not lie flat on your back at any time during your pregnancy as it impedes circulation to your baby.

Modify your work commute by reducing the amount of standing and driving. Ask someone on the bus, subway or train to get up and give you a place to sit down. When you are on the job, make a conscious effort to sit as often as possible. Cut down on the physical efforts you make – lifting, carrying, and so on. Avoid noise and fatigue as much as you can and try to fit in at least two rest periods during the day. Lie down to rest, preferably on your left side to increase blood flow to your heart. Ask your employer to help you modify your work environment to reduce the number of hours you work, or devise a compromise between working at home and at the office.

Emily, a thirty-five-year-old nurse and mother of two preschoolers, worked twelve-hour shifts every Saturday and Sunday in the emergency room of a large urban hospital during her last pregnancy. The working conditions were noisy and stressful; she rarely got to sit down for more than a few minutes, usually didn't finish a meal, and frequently had to help lift patients who were unconscious or couldn't move themselves. At 32 weeks gestation, Emily went into labor during a particularly stressful shift. She was admitted to the hospital and given medications to try to stop her contractions, but within a few hours she gave birth. Her son weighed four pounds at birth and spent a week in newborn intensive care and another two weeks in the newborn nursery.

Beth, a thirty-seven year old professional baker, was pregnant with her second child. Her first pregnancy was fifteen years ago, when she was in college. Divorced from the father of her first child and remarried, both she and her life were very different this second time around. First, she was older and got much more tired by the end of the day than she remembered feeling with her first pregnancy. Second, her daily work was much more stressful and demanding then when she was in college and her work environment was frequently hot and noisy. To reduce her risks of premature delivery, Beth took several important preventative steps. She cut down the number of hours she worked per day from eight to six; she cut down the number of days she worked from five to four; she changed her work hours to when the kitchens were less busy, to reduce stress and exposure to noise; and she sat instead of standing whenever possible. Beth worked this modified schedule for the last eight weeks, then stayed home for the last two weeks of her pregnancy. At 39 weeks gestation, she gave birth to a healthy 7 pound 6 ounce baby girl.

Lifestyle changes are completely under your control. Stop smoking and drinking. Don't take any drug–not even a vitamin or an aspirin – without checking with your health team. Reduce your caffeine intake to fewer than 300 milligrams per day. Follow medical guidelines regarding recreational exercise. You'll soon be able to get back in shape after the birth; don't push yourself to exercise vigorously now.

Eating right is the single most important thing you can do for your baby. Fasting, or going without food for prolonged periods, has been associated with the onset of labor. When the blood sugar level drops as a result of fasting, the body compensates by releasing free fatty acids from adipose tissue which can stimulate uterine contractions. Fasting also causes a release of the catecholamine stress hormones, which also lead to uterine contractions. It is particularly important, therefore, that during pregnancy you eat frequently, every two to three hours, and include breads, fruits or rice or pasta, all of which contain carbohydrates, at each meal.

Iron-deficiency anemia is associated with a 2.5-fold increased risk of prematurity and nearly a 3-fold increased risk of low birth weight. Many women have low iron stores, caused most often by heavy monthly menstrual periods. Other causes of low iron stores can include dieting, especially when meats are excluded, bleeding ulcers or hemorrhoids, and the frequent use of iron-binding medications, such as antacids. Tea and coffee can also contribute to the development of iron deficiency. Foods rich in easily absorbed iron include meat, fish and poultry.

Water is a substance vital to life, second in importance only to oxygen.

Like many people, you may not consider water an important part of your diet, but it certainly is! Water plays an important role in regulating body temperature through the evaporation of moisture from the skin and lungs. The loss of 1 to 2 percent of total body water triggers thirst, the loss of 10 percent constitutes a serious health hazard, and a 20 percent loss can result in death. During your pregnancy you should be drinking at least six to eight glasses of water a day. This amount is important to help prevent kidney infections, as well as to prevent dehydration, another possible cause of premature uterine contractions.

Consuming 0.4 milligrams of folic acid per day from at least one month prior to becoming pregnant through the first three months of pregnancy can reduce many birth defects. Make sure you're getting enough iron and calcium, from foods or supplements, and choosing the best vitamin supplement for your needs. Eat small mini-meals throughout the day and evening as you are continuing to nourish your placenta and your baby every moment of the day. We are what we eat, and that goes for your baby too!

There are many things we do not know about prematurity. Sadly, prematurity cannot be completely prevented. However, identifying and modifying your personal risk factors are the best ways to improve your chances of having a healthy, full-term pregnancy.

3

Third Month

Above all, enjoy your pregnancy. It's a very special time in your life and it doesn't last long.

Begin now to nap at least once a day. Even thirty minutes a day on your lunch hour will make a difference in your emotional and physical health.

Keep a pregnancy journal if you like. Write your feelings, body changes, thoughts and dreams down. A journal will help you to express yourself and will make interesting reading for your future generation.

Be aware of expectations – yours, the father's, your family's, your doctor's. Each party will have a different idea of how the next few months will proceed. Talk over your feelings in detail with each interested party. This may help to dispel any differences in expectations. For example, if you plan to work up to your eighth month, but your partner expects you to work to the end of your pregnancy, you have different expectations. Working out these details before your baby arrives will make your transition to a family smoother.

Plan to eat several small meals a day instead of your usual three. Large meals at breakfast, lunch and dinner do not tend to stay well on your stomach. Eating small meals and having healthy snacks in between is a much better format. Continue to have mini-meals when your baby arrives and especially when you are breastfeeding.

Keep snacks in your car or desk. Dried apricots or prunes will increase the iron in your blood. Granola bars can give you instant energy and fruit will keep your bowels moving. Your baby and placenta draw nutrition continually from your body, so keep your body well nourished with good foods at all times.

Have a quick snack before you go out if you know you will have to wait a long time before eating.

Connecting With Your Baby

There is good evidence in support of intrauterine bonding, written and researched by Dr. Thomas Verny in his book, *The Secret Life of The Unborn Child*. Your love relationship with your baby begins in your womb and expands after birth. Awareness that your baby has an emotional as well as a physical life can help you to feel more connected as you go about your daily activities. Your baby can hear, see, feel and touch while in the womb so that any interaction you choose, like holding your baby in your womb, talking to your baby, playing music to your baby and even just thinking or talking to your baby helps you both to connect at a deeper level.

Health Danger Signals

If at any time during your pregnancy you feel that either you or your baby are in any danger, go immediately to your doctor or nearest hospital. Do not delay. Always follow your intuition and instincts in regard to your health and your baby's health. Some signals of danger include early contractions, leaking amniotic fluid, any bleeding or spotting, fainting, seeing black spots, cramping or any marked change you may see in your pregnancy that you feel is not normal. Talking to a birth professional at the first sign of a problem will help to turn things around as quickly as possible if there is a problem. Trust your intuition if it is telling you that something is wrong.

Natural Remedies for High Blood Pressure

High blood pressure is a serious concern to pregnant women. If you have any symptoms of seeing spots before your eyes, swelling of your face, hands or feet, feeling faint or just feeling unwell, have your blood pressure checked immediately. Should you have a problem with your blood pressure, you might want to increase the protein in your diet. Increasing the calcium in your diet can also help. Take the calcium at bedtime with a small amount of food as the biggest drain on calcium stores is when you are sleeping.

If you are experiencing blood pressure problems you must consult a health professional immediately for your sake and your baby's sake. Homeopathic treatments can also assist greatly with this problem. Continue salting your food. New studies are showing salt is critically important during pregnancy. Add either chelated or a liquid calcium supplement to your diet immediately. Organically grown vegetables will also add to your calcium stores, which are being used on a daily basis for your baby.

Pre-Eclampsia – The Hidden Threat of Pregnancy

Pre-eclampsia, metabolic toxemia of late pregnancy (MTLP) has caused life threatening problems for mothers. Dr. Thomas H. Brewer has worked with over 7,000 pregnant women providing prenatal care and has found that mothers who eat a protective balanced diet including half a quart of milk, two eggs and two portions of fish or lean meat (with salt to taste) daily can prevent eclampsia. Women following this program did not have a single case of eclampsia, no toxic abruptio placentae and no maternal death. Dr. Brewer also mentions that, so far, United States and Canadian health professionals still insist the cause of eclampsia is unknown.

Preventing a High-Risk Pregnancy

Dr. Thomas H. Brewer's simple common-sense message to mothers for preventing a high-risk pregnancy is to eat for two, three or four. Avoid all drugs, street and doctor prescribed. Salt to taste, water to thirst, exercise and rest when tired.

Dr. Joel Wallach, BS, DVM, MD, Nobel Prize Nominee, one of the world's leading nutrition experts, has found that over 98% of all animal and human deaths are now caused by nutritional deficiencies. Lack of calcium alone causes over 180 diseases in modern man. Pregnancy draws calcium from all of your stores. Many common pregnancy problems like intense food cravings, high blood pressure, bleeding gums, muscle cramping, morning sickness, low blood sugar, chronic lower-back pain and other discomforts are caused by a lack of calcium, selenium, chromium, copper, and the fifty other minerals are just as important, or more important, than vitamin supplements during pregnancy. Before you reach for a glass of milk, Tums or calcium tablet, you should know your body will absorb less than 10% from any of these sources. Proper mineral nutritional support should include a liquid form of minerals known as colloidal minerals. These liquid minerals are over 98% absorbable by you and your baby.

Combining the expertise of these two physicians can help assure you of having a healthy pregnancy and a healthy baby.

Natural Remedies for Constipation

Being unable to move your bowels on a regular basis can cause your blood pressure to rise dangerously high. Make certain your prenatal vitamins are low in iron to prevent constipation. If you are finding constipation is still a problem, increase the amount of raw fruits and vegetables in your diet.

Excerpted from *Take Charge of Your Body,* Dr. Carolyn DeMarco, 7th Edition, 1997.

During pregnancy your body produces a hormone called progesterone. This hormone has the effect of relaxing the smooth muscles of your small and large intestines. Thus food passes through your intestines more slowly. Also your growing uterus may press on and displace the intestines. Another major factor contributing to constipation is taking iron supplements.

1.   Drink plenty of fluids. Some suggest six to eight glasses of fluid a day. This fluid should consist of pure water, fruit juice or herbal teas.
2.   Eat food that is high in fibre such as fresh fruit, vegetables and whole grains. Cut down or eliminate red meat, which is very constipating. Chicken or fish can be eaten instead.
3.   One to two tablespoons of unsulphured blackstrap molasses in warm

water once or twice a day is a reliable old remedy for constipation. Molasses is also high in iron and trace minerals. Be sure to brush your teeth well after you take molasses.

4. Some women find that drinking eight ounces of prune juice daily keeps their bowels moving.

5. Unrefined bran can be taken daily with whole grain cereal.

6. Ground flax seed, two tablespoons in water twice a day or metamucil without sugar are two mild laxatives that can be taken safely throughout pregnancy.

7. Discontinue your iron tablets or switch to a less constipating brand or a liquid iron, like Floradix, available in health food stores. I also have had great success with NutriChem iron, which is completely non-constipating.

8. Walk or do some type of physical exercise every day. This promotes regular bowel movements.

9. For some, changing position while sitting may help. For example, the backless chairs, where your knees are lower than your hips.

10. When you are pregnant, the timing of your bowel movement changes. Never sit on the toilet for long periods of time or strain during bowel movements as this can contribute to the development of hemorrhoids. If the stool is not passing easily, force yourself to get off the toilet and go about your businesss until you really have to go and the stool will then pass more easily.

Drugs

Stay away from all over-the-counter headache remedies, cold medications, aspirin, or anything that has not been prescribed by your doctor. If you have a persistent cold that is wearing you down, go to your neighborhood health food store or see a homeopathic doctor for a natural remedy.

Tobacco

Stop smoking. Many birth defects have been linked to the chemicals in tobacco smoke. Cigarette smoking cuts the amount of oxygen available in the maternal blood, which directly affects the growth of fetal tissue.

Alcohol

Do not drink alcohol during your pregnancy. Each day another part of your baby is growing or being developed; even one drink can stop or slow down development. Make a commitment to yourself and your baby to eliminate alcohol from your diet. Fetal Alcohol Syndrome can happen at any stage during your pregnancy if you drink alcohol. Any alcohol you drink is transmitted directly into your womb and concentrates in your baby's brain tissue, leaving your baby with permanent, irreversible organic brain damage. If you are unable to stop drinking on your own, seek professional help immediately.

What You Need to Know Before You Have Your Baby: Leading New Discoveries on Nutrition During Pregnancy

Excerpted from Alternative Medicine: The Definitive Guide, *by The Burton Goldberg Group, 1995.*

It is important to the health of both mother and fetus that the mother eats a well-balanced and varied diet. Fresh fruits and vegetables, whole grains, legumes, beans, and fish are essential. Limit refined sugars, processed foods, and saturated fats. Organically grown produce, meats, and poultry are preferable. However, if produce is not organic, it should be washed to remove as much of the agricultural chemicals as possible.

Most physicians recommend eating plenty of dairy products during pregnancy, due to their calcium and protein content. Other doctors are more wary about suggesting dairy as a mainstay of a pregnant woman's diet. Lendon Smith, MD, a pediatrician and author of several books on children's nutrition, explains, "Many babies will develop a milk sensitivity before they are born because the mother followed the obstetrician dictum: 'Drink a quart of milk every day so the baby will get the calcium.' If a mother is already sensitive to dairy products and takes in milk, cheese, and ice cream, she may not be absorbing the calcium from those foods she is ingesting." Foods such as nuts, soybean products, such as tofu and soy milk, and goat milk products provide alternative sources of protein. Seaweed, green vegetables, and a mixture of sunflower, sesame, and pumpkin seeds are alternatives for calcium. No one food, including dairy, should be eaten on a daily basis, says Dr. Smith, as this practice increases an individual's chance of developing a food sensitivity. Contrary to popular belief, a well-chosen vegetarian diet is healthy for a pregnant woman. Vegetarians who consume no animal products at all, including dairy and eggs, should use a B12 supplement.

Eating five to six small, nutrient-dense meals a day is a sensible idea. Restricting weight gain, which was very popular twenty years ago, was thought to ease a woman's labor. We now know that this is not necessarily so. New guidelines, issued in June 1990 by the Institute of Medicine in Washington, D.C. recommend increased weight gains for healthy pregnant women. The range of optimal weight gains depends on the weight of the mother early in pregnancy: twenty-eight to forty pounds for "underweight women", fifteen to twenty-five pounds for "overweight women", and a maximum of fifteen pounds for "obese women". These new guidelines, "reflect current interests in preventing low-birth weight babies and thus reduce the incidence of infant mortality and mental and physical retardation.

Pregnancy is not the time to diet. Dr. Linton offers a simple formula. "If you are eating a whole foods diet, drinking plenty of water, and getting adequate exercise such as walking or swimming, then the weight you gain in your pregnancy is appropriate."

Opinions vary on the amount of protein that is needed during pregnancy. Some experts advocate consuming even more protein than the Recommended Daily Allowance: "I think that dietary protein," says Dr. Birdsall, "is probably the most common nutrient deficiency in pregnancy." Pregnant women need seventy to one hundred grams of protein daily, which most people will not get with a normal diet. "These levels of protein," adds Birdsall, "help feed increasing blood volume and guard against complications during pregnancy, such as pre-eclampsia, a potentially dangerous condition characterized by high blood pressure, swelling and/or protein spilling into the urine."

Sodium is needed to maintain fluid balance and blood volume. For this reason, salt restriction is one common nutritional advisement that does not apply during pregnancy. Restricting sodium and using diuretics, once routine treatments to prevent pre-eclampsia and swelling, are not only unnecessary, but potentially harmful. It is best to use salt to taste.

Nutrition

Do not go on any calorie-reduced eating program while you are pregnant. The single most important thing you can do for your baby is to make sure you are eating well and eating often.

Our bodies are primarily composed of water and protein. Include protein with every meal. The most easily digested proteins are eggs, chicken, turkey and white fish.

Your personal need for water may change from day to day. If your urine is clear you can be assured that you have consumed enough water for that day.

A change in the food you purchase can make a vast difference in the health of your baby. If possible, purchase your fruits and vegetables organically. An organic tomato has 2,000 times more iron than a regular tomato. Organic lettuce has 60 times more calcium that regular lettuce.

Reduce the amount of sugar in your eating habits. Chocolate, pop, candy, ice cream and the like will stick to your thighs like gum. Junk food fills you up so that there is no room for good nutritious food.

Ask for water instead of pop with your food.

Ask for herbal non-caffeinated tea instead of coffee. Some of the best teas during pregnancy are red raspberry leaf tea, peppermint and ginger.

Wean yourself from regular coffee to half and half and then to decaffeinated coffee.

At parties, bring along a bottle of club soda without sodium, or try some non-alcoholic wine or beer. Or ask for a glass of water with a twist of lime or lemon.

Single and Pregnant

If you do not have a partner, think responsibly about what is best for you and your baby. Today mothers can have contact with adoptive families throughout the life of their child. A baby gives very little back to a parent initially and demands are on a twenty-four-hour clock. It is a tremendous burden of responsibility to bear alone. Keep in mind that when you are older you may have a greater wealth of resources to draw upon and remember that a woman's fertility can continue into her forties. You may want to look at adoption if you find yourself without a partner, take the time to discover all your options. Look in the yellow pages under adoption for the agencies operating in your area or in this guide in the Childbirth Resource Directory and interview two or three of the agencies to see if this option is right for you.

On the other hand, many women are raising their children alone in today's society by choice or circumstance. It is difficult, but possible. This is an intensely personal choice and one that each woman faces alone. There is no "right" answer or decision in this matter. Don't be pressured into making a quick decision. Take your time to look at all your options. If you choose to raise your baby on your own you can apply to the court for child support payments from the father of the baby if you feel he has an ability to provide them. Your local courthouse has a law library that is open to the public, and by studying child support cases you can do most of the legal work yourself. Child support cases are open to public viewing and there is usually one or two days a month set aside for these hearings, so you can watch the proceedings to get an idea of what happens. In Canada, be prepared to pay a one-time court filing fee of $200 or more. A hearing is then held to determine paternity and the ability of both partners to contribute financially to the child. You may wish to hire a lawyer for the final court date to insure that your case is properly heard.

Your Relationship

The first year with the first baby is considered the most hazardous time for every relationship. In this crucial adjustment year, husbands are more likely to feel insecure about being displaced by the baby, and their wives may feel abandoned, overwhelmed with feelings of inadequacy, fear or discouragement. Be aware that a baby will add more stress to your relationship and make sure that your relationship is strong and that both of you are in agreement on having a baby.

Both partners need an opportunity to ventilate frustrated and discouraged feelings in an accepting and supportive environment. Make sure you deal with issues as they arise and work together with your partner to find creative solutions to individual problems as they come up. Many couples report a decline in the satisfaction of their relationship after the birth of their first child. Have a plan to increase satisfaction in your relationship. You might want to contact an older couple with children to act as mentors or a marriage counsellor to help you to work through any rough spots.

Shopping Tips

Purchase good bras and maternity panties. A great bra for small to medium-size breasts is the sport type with hooks or snaps at front; they are made of Lycra elastic with wide shoulder straps. Sport-type bras keep everything in place and will stretch as you grow. If your breasts are larger make sure the shoulder strap on your bra is at least one inch across, as this will help in the distribution of weight and will stop the strap from cutting into your skin.

Cotton clothes absorb perspiration and are more comfortable than synthetics, especially in the summer months.

Go through your closet and put away all the clothing items you feel will be unsuitable for the months ahead. Purchase one or two pairs of black tights or leggings for casual wear. Look for shirts or sweaters in your closet that are large enough to cover your bottom to wear with your tights.

Plan to shop for maternity wear once a month rather than purchasing your entire wardrobe at once. Your needs will change as you progress along your pregnancy and shopping for a new article each month will give you the lift you need. Specialty pregnancy stores now have great selections of clothing for all occasions. Maternity stores are a recent development and will save you the frustration of having to collect your wardrobe from many different sources if you are pressed for time. If you were carrying extra pounds at the beginning of your pregnancy, you may want to check with Japanese Weekend Maternity Wear for their excellent selection in the "Abundant and Beautiful" line of pregnancy wear.

What You Need To Know Before You Have Your Baby: Electronic Monitoring Devices: Why You Don't Need Them

Excerpted from Silent Knife: Cesarean Prevention and Vaginal Birth After Cesarean, *Nancy Wainer Cohen and Lois J. Estner 1983*

There are two kinds of devices that are used to monitor labor, the Internal Fetal Monitor, IFM, and the External Fetal Monitor, EFM. In most labors neither one is safe or necessary.

First, the IFM. According to an article from the Feminist Health Works, this machine was originally designed as a diagnostic tool for the exceptionally high-risk labor, but it is now considered standard procedure for normal healthy labors.

The mother must lie flat on her back. We know by now this position in itself contributes to fetal distress; and that "except for hanging by the feet," it is the worst conceivable position for labor and delivery. It also requires artificial rupture of the bag of waters, another problematic procedure. Rupturing the membranes is necessary in this procedure so that two electronic catheters can be inserted into the vagina. One punctures and screws into the fetal scalp to monitor fetal well-being and the other lies between the fetus and the wall of the uterus to measure the pressure of the contraction.

The IFM can cause minor vaginal and cervical lacerations. Often the catheters become dislodged and have to be reinserted. The most consistent fetal complications to the baby are scalp bleeding, abscesses, and other bodily injuries. Sometimes the scalp electrode is misplaced and put into other places, such as an eyelid or a fontanelle. Ettner points out that this indwelling equipment provides a route for entry of bacteria from the vagina into the fluid with the results of infection and inflammation. It also can puncture the umbilical cord. It has been reported that cerebral spinal fluid has been caused to leak when the electrodes were incorrectly placed. It has been suggested by many researchers that the monitor causes the attendant to do more vaginal exams, which further increases the infection rate.

Several studies comparing the effectiveness of IFMs to listening to the baby's heart with a stethoscope or fetascope showed no difference between the groups. It is well known that monitoring is associated with increased cesarean section rates with no apparent improvement in infant outcome. Haverkamp's study shows a threefold increase in c-sections with no difference in infant outcomes. Thompson and Cohen also show a tripling of the cesarean rate that occurred with the popularization of IFM. Until the uncertainties of IFM are resolved, they say routine monitoring of low-risk births might itself be viewed as risky strategy. Drs. R. H. Paul and E. H. Hon tell us that the potential benefits of IFM are questionable. Its questionable accuracy is an important consideration, not to mention countless problems with misinterpretations of results.

The EFM in contrast consists of two straps placed around the mother's abdomen. One belt is a pressure gauge that monitors the pressure of the contractions. The other belt contains a device that measures the fetal heart rate. The machine translates information onto a sheet of paper that is excreted from a noisy machine next to the woman's bed. The woman is asked not to move from the bed as any movements can alter the readout.

Ettner concludes that such monitors show an entirely false sense of precision and that the information is inadequate as much as two-thirds of the time. Dr. John Patrick, of St. Joseph's Hospital, London Ontario, remarks that fetal monitors were in widespread use in hospitals before a study of their value had even begun. He believes that no one should have installed the machines until it was known whether or not they were of value, since there are risks involved. He also believes that doctors still don't know what the measurements on the machines mean, and this procedure has a 30% to 50% false positive result, (leading you to believe something is wrong when everything is fine). As presented in the paper, "Is Fetal Heart Rate Monitoring Worthwhile?" Patrick reports that one of the reasons the monitors are inaccurate is that the fetus moves and affects the measurements.

Banta and Thacker's article, "Electronic Fetal Monitoring: Is It of Benefit?" reports that careful review of the literature indicates little, if any increased benefit from EFM compared to manually monitoring the heartbeat. The risks, they say, are substantial. The National Institutes of Health task force on cesarean childbirth concluded that manually monitoring the heartbeat is an acceptable method of monitoring normal labor. Jarzembski does not feel that physicians are qualified to choose between different brands of monitors, much less to use them reliably. Ettner tells us that the benefits of electronic fetal monitoring do not outweigh the risks. Despite all this evidence, the trend toward universal EFM continues unabated. Banta and Thacker estimate that EFM involves an annual cost to our society (U.S.) of over $500 million dollars if the costs of cesarean sections and complications are included.

Mendelsohn, Ettner and others emphatically alert us to the fact that monitoring causes the distress it professes to detect. Murphy remarks that values from monitors are no better than simply tossing a fair coin. When you are forced to stay in bed and on your back, there's a good chance you'll end up with a cesarean, and a good chance it will be for failure to progress, FTP, or cephalopelvic disproportion, CPD.

Drugs During Childbirth: Is Any Drug Safe?

There is no drug that has been proven safe for a pregnant or laboring woman or her baby, yet the vast majority of women in our country take drugs during these times. It may be of interest that the FDA does not guarantee the safety of any drug, even those it has officially approved.

Drugs cause problems. To name a few, they cause nausea, confusion, raised or lowered blood pressure, and blurred vision – and all these conditions will also affect your baby. Brewer and Presser added that on drugs the patient can experience hallucinations, muscle spasms, a loss of urinary retention, headaches, tremors, and convulsions from toxic reactions. Drugs affect the uterus's ability to contract. We've lost count of the number of women who were sectioned for failure to progress, FTP, after a drug was administered.

Most of the effects of a particular drug are not known until it is too late. For example, Bendectin, a drug commonly prescribed for women with nausea during pregnancy, is now linked to several birth defects. According to Dowie and Marshall, Bendectin might very well be a teratogen, a drug or chemical that causes congenital malformation and defects in human and animal fetuses, like Thalidomide.

Brain disfunctions are now being linked to drugs given during labor. Fetal distress is a common reaction to these drugs. Maternal distress is equally common, since the drugs can cause irritability, depression, and "spacing out" in a woman as well as in her baby. Brewer and Presser say that the most damaging aspect of drug use during labor is that almost all drugs, when taken in amounts large enough to be effective in the mother, constitute an overdose for the baby. Most drugs work by depressing the central nervous system, and they can cause your baby to be limp, pallid, and unable to breathe on her own at birth. Drugged babies sometimes choke on their own mucus.

Susanne Arms, author of *Immaculate Deception*, writes "How many times must it be said? Drugs may permanently damage the baby. Any doctor who tells his patient that any drug used for any reason—including tranquilizers, sedatives, caudals, epidurals, saddle blocks, paracervical blocks, spinals, generals, or whatever—will not affect the baby is telling her an untruth: no drug has been proven not to affect the baby."

Abraham Lobin, writing in the *Journal of the American Medical Association,* reports, "Gestation and birth thus form an inexorable leveling mechanism; with the brain marred at birth, the potential of performance may be reduced from that of a genius to that of a plain child or less. The damage may be slight, imperceptible clinically, or it may spell the difference between brothers, one a dextrous athlete and the other an awkward child."

A study by Alan Gitzler at Downstate Medical Center in New York reports that a woman's natural pain tolerance is increased naturally before birth. Beta-endorphin, the brain's own morphine-like substance, is present in the human placenta as a natural antidote for the pain of childbirth. The endorphin system is responsible for this effect, and drugs can alter endorphin production. A preliminary study by Akil et al. at the University of Michigan showed that endorphin levels are six to seven times the normal level in pregnant women and jump even higher during birth. A study by Kimball suggests that elevated maternal endorphin levels evoke prolactin secretion which is related to maternal-infant bonding. According to Dr. Kimball, prenatal understanding and reassurance about the natural, powerful anesthetic effect of endorphins which can be obtained by active participation in labor provides incentive and confidence for expectant mothers.

Ultrasound: Valid Test or Smoke and Mirrors?

Ultrasound is seeing with sound, a complex technique for studying the inner organs of the body. Although it has not been proven safe, it is being used with increasing frequency in American obstetrics. In simple terms, high-frequency sound waves are beamed into the body. They bounce back from different surfaces and densities of various body organs. The echoing waves are duly measured and recorded.

Doris Haire, who is the director of the Association of Maternal Child Health in New York, has called ultrasound "the DES of tomorrow". DES was given to mothers up until the early 1970s to prevent miscarriage. It has since been proven it did not prevent miscarriage. But, much worse, twenty years after DES was first administered we all learned that it is associated with numerous reproductive abnormalities, high incidence of infertility and very high rates of cancer in the children whose mothers took it.

Diagnostic ultrasound has been around for decades, but has been widely used in pregnancy, birth and medical diagnosis for only the past seven to ten years. Children who were bombarded with ultrasound as fetuses are now reaching the ages of reading readiness and mental neurological evaluation. In fact, a current study funded by the FDA at the University of Colorado Medical Center, under the direction of Dr. Albert Haerkampk, is examining 1,600 children for reading or other learning disabilities as well as physical abnormalities that may be traced to ultrasound. Another study in Winnipeg, Canada, is following ten thousand exposed subjects.

Perhaps the most common use of diagnostic ultrasound is for gestational age determination. A determination of dates is possible with some accuracy only between the fourteenth and twentieth weeks of pregnancy, by measuring the biparietal diameter of the fetal head with ultrasound waves. However, most questions about dating seem to arise during the third trimester of a pregnancy, and as the weeks pass, measurements become increasingly inaccurate and useless because of variations in growth rates. Thus, all the ultrasound scans that are being done on third trimester women for dating purposes are, in our opinion, inappropriate, unnecessary, wasteful, improper, and worst of all, potentially harmful to the fetus. Even if a baby's due date is calculated in the sixteenth week by an ultrasound, that baby still could arrive three weeks early or three weeks late.

Some doctors order ultrasound scans routinely to determine if there is a low lying placenta. If this situation is present, they often insist upon a cesarean. The incidence of low-lying placentas seems to be on the increase; according to Esther Zorn, founder and president of the International Cesarean Prevention Movement, it may be that a low-lying placenta is something that exists fairly often and that it is just being discovered because of the use of ultrasound. Given time, she notes, the placenta often migrates up and away from the cervix. Another inappropriate use of ultrasound is for determination of the viability of a uterine pregnancy. If a woman begins to bleed or stain in her first trimester, she may miscarry or she may carry a healthy fetus to term and deliver a perfect baby.

The FDA has cautioned against the use of diagnostic ultrasound in the first trimester because of potential harm to the developing fetus. Yet many doctors have chosen to ignore the warnings. Some scans have shown viable, secure implantations but miscarriage occurred anyway. Ultrasound is unable to completely dispel anxiety, since the results may mean little or nothing in the overall scheme of that pregnancy; it should be carefully limited to such uses as early diagnosis of a suspected tubal pregnancy.

So, when you visit your physician, refuse the Doptone, which operates on the same system using a more powerful frequency as it is a hand-held ultrasound unit. You will be able to hear your baby's heartbeat at about the twentieth week with a stethoscope or fetascope. If diagnostic ultrasound is recommended, ask for full details: Why is it recommended? Would the results be absolutely accurate at this point in your pregnancy? Would the scan provide essential information that can not be gathered any other way and which would then determine resultant care? And what difference does it make if you already know your estimated due date?

4

Fourth Month

Motherhood will enable you to experience every aspect of who you are as a woman. You may find this experience the most challenging and rewarding position of your life.

Pregnancy affects your entire body and most of its functions. Don't be fooled into thinking that the only thing that changes is your tummy size.

Make sure your health team is available to talk to you about any aspect of pregnancy and childbirth. Pregnancy is not the time to be embarrassed to ask important questions about your health and the health of your baby. Ask questions. Being pregnant is at times confusing. Your health team will be able to tell you how your body will react to various things at various stages. No question is too small or stupid. Second or third pregnancies may be very different from the first.

Are you are having trouble getting your current OB to talk to you, answer your questions, make eye contact with you or smile at you? Think you may have to switch at this point? If you feel that you are getting an impersonal, assembly-line practice or that your birth plan may not be complied with, remember that it is never too late to switch. One mother switched her doctor four days past her due date and another changed during her labor.

Arrange now for a caregiver and a backup caregiver to assist you when you bring your new baby home. Many mothers feel that just getting through their pregnancy is the hard part; in reality the first thirty days after the birth of your child will continue to bring tremendous demands on your body and your hormonal system. Make sure you have the support necessary to heal completely from the birth when you bring your baby home. In many tribal societies the mothers rest and are cared for by their families for forty days after the birth of the child.

The Woman's Herb – The Remarkable Raspberry Leaf Tea

Although many people display allergic symptoms to strawberries, few cannot indulge in the winey fruit that ripens in the hottest part of the summer, the raspberry. The fruit is lovely, but the healthful properties in the leaves and root bark are so valuable, raspberry is known as the "Woman's Herb." Raspberry is a relative of the rose, famous for vitamin C in the rose hip. Raspberry leaves are rich in citric acid, malic acid, tartaric acid, citrate, malate and tartarate of iron, potassium and calcium, calcium and potassium chloride, sulphate and phosphate, pectin, fragrine, vitamins A, B, C, E and fructose. The action is astringent, tonic, refrigerant, parturient, hemostatic, anti-septic, anti-abortient, anti-gonorrheal, anti-leucorrheal and anti-malarial.

Regular drinking throughout pregnancy strengthens and tones tissues, helping contractions and checks hemorrhage during labor. A perfectly safe drink, unlike black tea or coffee, raspberry leaf tea also enriches milk and helps prevent miscarriage. Raspberry leaf tea has helped with painful menstruation and lessens an overabundant period. At menopause the adrenals are geared to take over as the ovaries gradually cease functioning. Many menopausal symptoms are caused by exhausted adrenals. Men with exhausted adrenals are well-advised to drink this tea as well. Red raspberry leaf tea with red clover, one or more cups daily for several months, promotes fertility in men and women, prevents postnatal depression and hypertension. Pour one cup boiling water over a teaspoon of dried leaves and let it steep at least 15 minutes. Drink and heal.

The Compleat Mother, the Magazine of Pregnancy, Birth and Breastfeeding, in their Spring 1996 issue reports that you can harvest wild or tame raspberry leaves in spring or mid-summer for maximum potency. Use them freshly picked, and dry them for storage away from the light. They dry nicely spread thinly on a cotton sheet hung hammock fashion from the ceiling. If you don't have access to a raspberry patch in your neighborhood, *The Compleat Mother* sells pure, fresh, organic raspberry leaf tea in a reusable tin (50 grams) for $8.00 Canadian and a Winter Supply (125 grams) for $10.00 Canadian. If you are ordering tea from *The Compleat Mother,* send along $22.00 for a one year bulk subscription (5 copies you can share with friends or health professionals) or $12.00 a year for a single subscription to their quarterly magazine. *The Compleat Mother* has an endearing and unending sense of humor and may be the best gift you buy for yourself and your new baby. Write to the office nearest you:

Compleat Mother – Canada, RR #3, Clifford, Ontario NOG lMO (519) 327-8785

Compleat Mother – USA, PO Box 209, Minot, ND 58702 (701) 852-2822

Compleat Mother – Netherlands, Kanaalstraat 54 HS, 1054 XK, Amsterdam

Compleat Mother – Australia, PO Box 610, Lulwyche, Queensland, Australia

Ambivalence

Some women are ambivalent about the baby they are carrying up until the last moment of their pregnancy. This doesn't have to be you. Your baby feels this emotion, and all other emotions you have while your baby is in your womb. This is the time to make up your mind about your pregnancy and to decide that you will do your best. Occasional thoughts of whether you have made the right decision will surface from time to time: this is normal. If these thoughts are constantly with you, review the reasons why you decided to have your baby. Be confident in your decision and in your ability to mother. An excellent book on emotions during pregnancy is *Transformation Through Birth* by Claudia Panuthos.

Exercising

Moderately exercising throughout your entire pregnancy will help you to keep your energy up and the extra weight down. Walking is still one of the best forms of exercise for a pregnant woman. A regular walking routine at your favorite time of day strengthens your thighs and hips, helping you to have a faster and easier childbirth. Regular exercise will also help you to deal with the emotional lows and highs of pregnancy and will give you the extra strength you will need for natural delivery of your baby. If you have never exercised before your pregnancy, start slowly and always stop before you are panting with exertion. Regular exercise will also improve your appearance and posture.

Regular exercise during your pregnancy can help you to have a faster and easier labor and delivery and walking helps your baby to turn more easily in your womb to a head-down position.

If you enjoy the water, specially designed water fitness classes for pregnancy can be found at most pools. Check out your city's Y.W.C.A.

There are specially designed exercise programs for pregnancy and a quick trip to the library will show you how to add something new to your exercise program while you are pregnant. Check with your health team before you begin.

Breastfeeding Your Baby

All most all women, around the world are breastfeeding again. Over 85% of Canadian women now breastfeed their babies. Breastfeeding is a learned skill, like riding a bike, skating, or driving a standard shift vehicle. This is a good time to begin reading up on breastfeeding, creating a support network, and understanding why your breast milk is so important for you and your baby.

Breastfeeding Facts

• Breastmilk is free.

- Breastfeeding is natural.
- Breastmilk is the best food available for your baby.
- Breastfeeding can create a strong bond of love and trust between you and your baby.
- Breastfed babies cry less often.
- Breastfed babies are calmer.
- Breastfed babies have colds of a much shorter duration, if any.
- Breastmilk can easily be frozen and stored for future use.
- Breastfed babies always receive the right amount of milk.
- Breastfed babies are easily taken with you.
- Breast size has no correlation to the amount of milk you produce.
- Breastfed babies are more secure.
- Breastfed babies have less gas.
- Breastmilk contains natural enzymes to help your baby easily digest each meal.
- Breastfeeding will not change the shape of your breasts, pregnancy can.
- Breastmilk provides all the nutrition your baby requires for the first six months of life. You do not have to supplement breast milk with any other food during this time. You will continue to produce breastmilk for as long as you choose to breastfeed.
- Some mothers are continuing to breastfeed their children into the second year and beyond to boost their children's immune systems. Breastmilk contains hundreds of antibodies that strengthen your baby's immune system.
- Breastmilk triggers the mothering hormone, prolactin, with every feeding causing you to feel more relaxed and attached to your new baby.
- Breastfed babies have better tooth and mouth development.
- Breastfeeding comforts you and your baby emotionally.
- Breastfeeding is convenient and economical.
- Breastfeeding can help you to have a lower incidence of breast cancer.
- Breastfeeding tones the muscles of your uterus and helps your body recover and recondition itself more rapidly.
- Breastmilk is ready when your baby is.
- Breastmilk changes its consistency throughout each feeding and will change to meet the needs of your baby as your baby grows.
- Breastmilk is the best milk for premature infants.
- Breastfeeding provides resistance to ear infections.
- Breastfeeding can help to prevent or forestall allergies and asthma.
- Breastmilk will cool or warm for your baby automatically.
- Breastmilk easily increases to meet the demands of your growing baby.
- Breastmilk is always sterile, clean and ready.

- Breastmilk can reduce celiac, crohns and colitis bowel diseases.
- Breastfeeding can reduce diabetes, pneumonia, obesity, meningitis, cirrhosis and lymphoma in your baby.
- Breastmilk is the best choice for every baby.

Secrets to Successful Breastfeeding

Is there a secret to successfully breastfeeding your baby? Maybe just one! Be prepared to spend all of your time breastfeeding! At least it may seem like this in the first two weeks. The key to the first month is to breastfeed whenever your baby is hungry, which usually means whenever she is awake. You may be breastfeeding every two hours during the first few days after your milk comes in. After the first few weeks you will have established your milk supply to suit your baby and you exactly and then you can relax. After the first month your baby will also become more proficient and each feeding becomes faster.

Many mothers are continuing their breastfeeding relationship with their babies when they return to their careers. You can breastfeed your baby in the mornings, the evenings and on the weekends. Once your breastfeeding has been established you will continue to produce breast milk. Some babies will change their feeding schedules around to take full advantage of you when you are available and have a heavier feeding demand during the evening rather than the day.

How do you relax when breastfeeding? It is hard to feel comfortable if you think everyone is watching you when you feed your baby. Find a quiet spot (in public or private), cover your baby and yourself with a large soft blanket and tune out your surroundings as best you can. This will take a little practice, but once you have it mastered, you will find being able to nurse anywhere, anytime is a real bonus.

When at a shopping mall you can go into any changing room in a department store, many malls now have special mother's rooms or you can go to your car for some peace and quiet for breastfeeding. Once you've had some practice you may find that you can easily breastfeed anywhere without attracting any attention at all. Just make sure you are pulling up your top rather than undoing the buttons to keep your chest covered. At a party ask to use an empty bedroom if you like. In your home set up a private space with your rocker and footstool and a small table for books, telephone, a glass of juice or water and high energy snacks. Let everyone at home know that this is your spot for breastfeeding and that you will defend your territory.

Wearing nursing-accessible clothing is a must. Two-piece outfits work best; pants and a T-shirt, a skirt and blouse, tights and long sweaters. It is difficult to breastfeed your baby in the wrong clothing. Remember to wear two-piece outfits to bed. It can get cool in the middle of the night so keep a housecoat at the foot of your bed or within easy reach.

People ask a lot of questions when you are breastfeeding. "Does it hurt?" "Aren't you embarrassed?" "Wouldn't a bottle be easier?" Try to answer them honestly and openly. They are just curious. Answer these questions with a smile and tell whoever asks why you've chosen to breastfeed. Satisfy their curiosity. After all, the more people who are educated about breastfeeding, the more support there will be for everyone.

How do you keep siblings entertained while breastfeeding? Breastfeeding is especially time-consuming in the first few weeks, and an older brother or sister may feel left out of the loop. One of the best things you can do while breastfeeding is to read to the older children. Have the older child sit beside and turn the pages when you "beep." This also has a calming effect on your baby, as the older child is not running about pleading for attention.

How do you keep your partner involved if you are doing all the feeding? Let your partner know that you will be expressing milk and freezing it to create a milk bank that any member of the family can access to feed the baby. In the first few weeks after the birth of your baby you will have an abundance of milk, making this an excellent time to start your own milk bank. Have your partner choose his favorite baby task and have him be in charge of that activity. Set up a special time in the evening for them to enjoy their activity or task together.

Sleeping when your baby sleeps is a tried and true method to combat exhaustion. Doing housework during this period will add to the natural tiredness you may be feeling. Save the housework for when your baby is up and alert; you can easily place your newborn in a portable infant seat for company while you go about your tasks. In the first few months you must guard your energy, and having one or two short naps during the day or early evening will recharge your batteries. Ask for help with the laundry, cooking, shopping and whatever else you need.

Older children can spend quiet time in their rooms every day. Keep in mind that this quiet time may sometimes be at odd hours, but it is quiet time, nonetheless. If they are old enough, they can understand that quiet time is not always just after lunch, but may come at 2:30 when the baby's sleeping. Set the kitchen timer to wake you up in 45 minutes so that the older child is not left in their room for too long.

Breastfeeding your baby can make you hungry and thirsty. Make up a tray of mini-muffins, healthy cookies or fruit. Something you can grab (with one hand) in the middle of the night. A shot of milk, juice or water helps to fight dehydration, which you may feel at night. Keep these items within easy reach. Snacking while you breastfeed your baby can also assist in fighting fatigue. Keep bottles of water in the car and one in your purse.

Consider breastfeeding for at least a one-year period to give your baby an immune advantage. Many babies are developing intolerances and allergies to dairy and one quarter of these babies are also intolerant to soy milk. Finding an alternative food source for a six-month old allergic baby is almost impossible.

Shopping Tips

Find a maternity shop that rents clothing for the office and special occasions. Look for an elegant, formal outfit that you may need to wear in the months to come. Dark, solid colors without prints, patterns or buttons will make you feel less conspicuous, and you will look and feel more elegant.

Look for a second-hand pregnancy consignment in your area under Clothing in your Yellow Pages directory. Great prices for clothing you will only be wearing a few months at the most.

Go to the Plus-Size shops for maternity wear like Additionelle. Look for oversize tops in solid colors to go with your tights or dress pants to stretch your wardrobe dollar further.

During your last trimester your feet may swell. Buy any new shoes at least a half size larger with room to stretch. Easy Spirit shoes are excellent dress shoes for pregnancy.

Purchase a blazer or suit jacket in a size two or three sizes larger than you usually wear. Make sure that you purchase this in a solid color so that you can wear it with most of your outfits. You may be able to wear this for many months and it will help you feel more put together when you dress for work or the office.

What You Need to Know Before You Have Your Baby: Breech Presentation: Medical Fashion Changes

Henci Goer has compiled an outstanding research report that teaches you how to easily understand obstetric literature. She shows that midwifery and out of hospital births are scientifically valid and are just as likely, if not more likely to result in a healthy baby and mother. She also shows how the routine use of technology can do harm. Henci provides scholarly and detailed evaluations of the many controversial interventions and issues involved in obstetrical care. Reading this book will give you a clear look into the field of obstetrics without the bias of the belief that a procedure is valid and necessary due to its current popularity.

Henci is an ASPO-certified Lamaze teacher and doula. A medical writer for many years, she has written numerous pamphlets and magazine articles for childbirth professionals and for expectant couples. She is a member of Birth Work's Board of Advisors and *Childbirth Instructor Magazine's* Editorial Advisory Board. Her book *Obstetric Myths Versus Research Realities: A Guide to the Medical*

Literature, has garnered uniformly positive reviews, and several midwifery schools have adopted it as a textbook. In 1993, the National Association of Childbearing Centers (NACC) gave her its Media Award, and in 1995, ASPO/Lamaze honored her with its President's Award in recognition of her book. Henci Goer is married and has three children.

Excerpted from Obstetric Myths Versus Research Realities *Henci Goer, 1995.*

Medical fashion changes. In the past some doctors deliberately reached inside at the delivery to turn head down babies breech and pull them out feet first. Now most doctors believe that vaginal breech (baby presents buttocks or feet first) birth is so dangerous that it should not be permitted. Breech babies do suffer higher mortality and morbidity rates, but the two cures – external cephalic version (turning the baby by manipulating it from the outside), (ECV), and universal cesarean section–are not so straightforward a cure as they would seem.

Cephalic version, CV, is an old technique. Anthropologist Brigitte Jordan (1984) documents that midwives and doctors throughout the world have long practiced it with few complications. But always they have stressed that problem-free success depends on a gentle, patient manipulator and a comfortable, relaxed mother.

Unfortunately, some not-so-gentle doctors, using general anesthesia and brute force, caused placental abruptions (detachment from the uterine wall), hemorrhages, and fetal distress. . . Some babies died. Predictably, doctors condemned ECV instead of their technique. Because cesarean for breech is all but universal, despite the rarity of breech presentation, it is the third most common reason for cesarean section (VanTuinen and Wolfe 1992).

Does cesarean section improve breech outcomes? The major reasons why breech babies have more problems than vertex babies have nothing to do with birth route. Breech babies are more likely to be premature or growth retarded. They are more likely to have congenital anomalies, genetic defects, or neuromuscular deficits or problems such as hip dysplasia or cerebral palsy (Claussen and Nielsen 1988; Hytten 1982). This is because size, weight, shape, and normal movements guide the baby into the head-down position. In most cases vaginal breech birth did not cause the problem, and cesarean section will not cure it. . .

The woman with a breech fetus should try self-help strategies to turn it starting in the eighth month, then ECV, and if ECV fails, she should seek evaluation for vaginal breech birth from someone experienced, ideally someone whose practices promote spontaneous birth. Optimal management for a preterm or twin breech or when no one is experienced with vaginal breech is unclear. Women should insist on a sonogram to rule out anomalies incompatible with life before agreeing to a cesarean. And whatever she decides, she must understand that no matter what is done (or not done), good outcome cannot be guaranteed – and that includes delivering the baby by cesarean.

Gestational Diabetes: Fact or Fiction?

In normal pregnancy, certain hormones make extra glucose available to the fetus by preventing the mother's insulin from doing its normal job of transporting glucose out of her bloodstream into her own cells. This insulin-suppressant effect increases as pregnancy advances. . .

During the 1960s and 1970s doctors began studying the effects of glucose intolerance in pregnant women; however, the studies were poorly designed (Goer 1991). Sometimes they selected women for glucose testing on the basis of previous poor pregnancy outcome or risk factors in the current pregnancy and then compared outcomes with the general population. Some mixed in known prepregnant diabetics. They often failed to account for confounding factors. In short, the studies thoroughly obscured the true risk of subdiabetic glucose intolerance in pregnancy. . . [Nonetheless] the results convinced researchers that they had discovered a serious problem, and in 1979 they convened the first of what became a series of exponentially larger international conferences (Metzger 1991a). . .

Articles about the diagnosis and treatment of gestational diabetes (GD) almost always begin with a litany of the supposed dangers of untreated GD: perinatal death, congenital anomalies, macrosomia, neonatal hypoglycemia, hyperbilirubinemia (neonatal jaundice), other neonatal metabolic abnormalities, and maternal hypertension. Reducing the incidence of macrosomia is also supposed to reduce the number of instrumental and cesarean deliveries as well as birth injuries and asphyxia.

Accordingly, women diagnosed as gestational diabetics will find themselves plunged into anything from an unpleasant experience to a living nightmare, depending on their degree of glucose intolerance and their doctors' whim (Gillmer et al. 1986). They may have blood tests anywhere from weekly to several times a day, dietary and calorie restriction, extra doctor visits, prenatal surveillance and weight estimate tests (all of which have high false-positive rates), insulin injections, prenatal hospitalization, induction of labor, and/or repeated glucose monitoring during labor. (Knopp et al. 1991; Jovanovic-Peterson and Peterson 1991; Coustan 1991; Dickinson and Palmer 1990; Chez et al. 1989; Reed 1988; Landon and Gabbe 1988; Board et al. 1986; ACOG 1986). The odds of cesarean – both scheduled and in labor – are greatly increased compared with nongestational diabetics carrying babies of the same weight (Goldman et al. 1991; Acker, Sachs, and Friedman 1985). The infants of GD mothers may be subjected to repeated heel sticks to determine blood glucose, removed to nurseries for observation, or fed glucose water, which interferes with establishing breastfeeding (Hod et al. 1991). . .

The fact is that only those who were true diabetics prior to pregnancy or those few whose pregnancies have tipped them into a true diabetic state benefit from special care. Beyond that, women who are overweight should try to achieve normal weight before pregnancy, because maternal weight bears the strongest relationship with infant birth weight and glucose tolerance. Women with subdiabetic glucose intolerance during pregnancy should eat a diet low in simple sugars and high in complex carbohydrates and fiber, and health permitting, they should exercise moderately and regularly. . . This, of course, is advice that would profit any pregnant woman. As for GD, after reviewing the literature Hunter and Keirse (1989) say, "Except for research purposes, all forms of glucose tolerance testing should be stopped."

Premature Rupture of Membranes At Term: New Answers

Myth: Once membranes are ruptured, the baby must be born within 24 hours or infection sets in. Reality: "By waiting 24 hours, avoiding cervical examination, and allowing a reasonable latent phase of labor. . . we believe that the increase in cesarean section rates with induction can be minimized."(Garite 1985).

In the 1960s a flurry of papers on the infectious hazards of prolonged rupture of the fetal membranes led to the 24-hour rule: once membranes rupture the baby must be delivered within 24 hours. In order to ensure time enough for labor, this meant inducing any woman who did not begin spontaneous labor within a few hours of membrane rupture, augmenting slowly progressing labors with oxytocin, and performing cesarean sections on those for whom delivery was not imminent by 24 hours postrupture. Babies born after or close to the 24-hour limit were likely to be subjected to a septic workup to determine if the neonate was infected, which included drawing blood and often a spinal tap.

This aptly named "aggressive approach" was enthusiastically embraced by obstetricians, who expressed delight at having a rationale for intervening – although, in what is surely unintentional irony, they did not like the word aggressive. They feared it might give a negative impression because aggression means "a first or unprovoked attack or an attack of hostility" (Russell and Anderson 1962). Concerns about potentially high cesarean section rates and the observation that infections were rare when no vaginal exams were performed were brushed aside (Russell and Anderson 1962), and by the early 1970s, the 24-hour rule had become the standard of practice in term pregnancies. Aggressive management did, in fact, lead to high cesarean rates for failed induction or fetal distress, but this was considered preferable to the lethal perinatal infections that would surely result from doing nothing. . .

The relationships between rupture of membranes, labor, and infection are more complex than the doctors of the 1960s (or for that matter, the decades since) believed. Cooperstock, England, and Wolfe (1987) studied the association between time of rupture and time of day and found that not all cases of PROM are alike. Women who began spontaneous labor within a day or so after membrane rupture were highly likely to have membranes rupture late at night. Women with infected membranes (chorioamnionitis) did not show this circadian rhythm. Neither did women who were not infected but who did not begin labor within that time frame. Observing that labor onset shows the identical circadian pattern, the authors theorized that in the first case, hormones regulating the onset of labor were probably responsible. The second case suggests that infection precipitated membrane rupture. In the third case, some as yet unknown mechanism appeared to be at work.

Their study illuminates the problems of PROM. It explains why inductions often fail: women whose uteruses are not primed for labor – that is, women in categories two and three – will not labor effectively no matter how much oxytocin is given (Steer, McCarter, and Beard 1985). It explains the seeming relationship between length of time postrupture and infection. Women in the second category (comprising very few term pregnancies) have an incipient infection. They are not ready to labor and will have a long latency period, which will allow that infection to blossom. In women of the third category, vaginal exams and internal monitoring start infective processes that, as with the second case, have time to take hold because these women, too, have a long latency period. Finally, it explains why almost all studies of PROM management at term done since the 1960s show major benefits for expectant management (watching and waiting) in women with no signs of infection: women who are not infected are not likely to develop infections – provided people keep their fingers and monitoring devices out of the vagina and will do best if left alone.

The fact is not only does leaving women alone do best for most women, but standard management could hardly do worse if it were intentionally designed that way. Standard management causes infections and fetal distress, the very things it is supposed to prevent. Vaginal exams and internal monitoring start infections. Induction leads to vaginal exams, internal monitoring, fetal distress, and c-sections, which themselves have much higher infection rates. .

Local application of prostaglandin gel is rapidly gaining prominence as an alternative to waiting for labor, but as we shall see, it does no better than expectant management [watching and waiting] at minimizing cesareans; it sometimes does worse; and it introduces risks. . . The 2% to 4% of women who do not proceed to spontaneous labor for whatever reason within a day or so (Duncan and Beckley 1992) are likely to prove problematic whatever is done.

Induction is no panacea, even for this tiny minority. . .

[Watching and waiting] for 24 hours and probably longer is safe. Few women or babies develop clinical infections [during this period]. Waiting 24 hours before inducing allows 60% to 95% of women to start labor spontaneously. . . PROM can be managed on an outpatient basis.

Her closing words are as follows, "My critique of obstetric care . . . derives from a commonly held feminine perspective that would reclaim childbearing as an empowering act, one in which women would be cherished, nourished, supported, celebrated, and respected."

Henci Goer goes on to cover Cesarean, Vaginal Birth After Cesarean, Epidurals, Inductions, Electronic Fetal Monitoring, Episiotomies, Routine IVs Versus Eating and Drinking in Labor, Amniotomy, Freestanding Birth Centers, Midwives, Home Birth and the Nature of Evidence: Why the Gap Between Belief and Reality, with the same degree of thoroughness and logic.

You can find out more about Obstetric Myths Versus Research Realities *by visiting her web site at http://www.efn.org/~djz/birth/obmyth/. There is an order form at the site or you may write to her at 970 Buckeye Court, Sunnyvale, CA 94086 USA. Henci's next book will be called* The Thinking Woman's Guide to a Better Birth. *Write to the above address to receive advance notice of this next publication. Copies of* Obstetric Myths Versus Research Realities *can also be purchased directly through the above address.*

5

Fifth Month

Be prepared for many new emotions and dreams. Hormonal fluctuations will affect every aspect of your emotions. When you feel like crying, cry. If you find your anger surfacing use it to move forward with your life. Explain your feelings, as they come up, to your baby if you like. It is also comforting to talk them out with your partner and friends.

Make fruit your bedtime snack. You will find that fruit will satisfy your appetite and your need for extra nutrition. Fruit adds fiber, quenches your thirst, and will help you to have fewer trips to the bathroom during the night.

Read the breastfeeding section in this book during this month. Go to the library and watch breastfeeding videos. The more you know about breastfeeding now, the easier you will breastfeed your baby. Plan to attend a breastfeeding clinic in your eighth or ninth month of pregnancy. Call the La Leche number listed in the Childbirth Resource Directory to find a breastfeeding support group right in your neighbourhood. You will be welcomed with open arms while you are pregnant and after. In the support group you will hear of common challenges in breastfeeding and common solutions. Often any challenges can be cleared up with a phone call or a quick meeting. Just knowing where to direct your inquiries can give you peace of mind.

If you experience pain from your stomach muscles stretching as your baby grows, lean forward all the way while sitting to relieve the pressure on these muscles, whenever you feel the stretch.

Rock your baby in the womb. Place both hands on either side of your stomach and slowly breath in and out. You can do this first thing in the morning or last thing at night to relax both of you. Your baby will feel the soothing warmth of your hands and will always be comforted by this time together.

A woman carries her birth experience with her for rest of her life. The childbirth process is not simply a means to the end of the pregnancy. When planning your childbirth remember that this will be the most important day of your baby's life as well. What matters most is a healthy baby and mother.

Managing Fear of Labor And Delivery

You may have fears of labor that come up from time to time. Instead of focusing on the unknown, focus instead of the joy you will feel as you gaze into your baby's eyes and how your baby will feel against your breast as you feed your baby for the first time. Often mothers find the birth of their second child much easier than the first baby as there is less fear of the unknown. When the time comes for your child to be born nature takes over and you may be surprised at the efficiency of your body during the birth process.

Talk through your fears of pregnancy, labor and delivery and parenthood with your partner, your doctor and good friends. It will always help to ease your mind when you verbalize your concerns to others. Have faith in the natural process of childbirth, read as much as you can about childbirth, attend an informative prenatal class and plan to have professional labor support with you during your labor and delivery. Occasionally our fears are replayed in life. Decide what you are most afraid of, whether it be cesarean, dealing with pain during labor, episiotomy, stalled labor, or whatever may be concerning you personally and read everything you can on how to deal with that situation that you are most concerned with. Talk over solutions to any of your concerns with your health team.

The Wise Women

Here are some more letters from Open Season – A Survival Guide for Natural Childbirth and Vaginal Birth After Cesarean, VBAC in the 90's *Nancy Wainer Cohen, 1991, on why midwifes are becoming the first choice for many women in Canada and the United States.*

"I have an unfaltering confidence in birth, in a woman's ability to give birth, and in myself as a practitioner. No woman has ever looked in my eyes and seen doubt and that unfailing encouragement is what helps to get stuck babies out. This is what I love. I will always be reborn in midwifery, each day and with each birth." Meg

"You know, there is always so much more to learn. When I observed other midwives I saw them sitting on their hands and being supportive. I learn to sit on my hands, to trust, more and more each day. A woman with four previous classical cesareans wanted a homebirth. Everyone thought she was crazy and that I would be even crazier for attending her. My heart said, 'Do it. It will be fine. I always listen to my heart. It never lies to me." Mary

"Every time I saw an OB cut a woman's perineum, I felt my own was being cut. Finally I said 'No more!' I put my hand in front of the OB's knife and said, 'Cut off my fingers first." Carolyn

"I learned early that patience is a virtue. Perhaps it comes from growing up in a large family, I don't know. Some women are just in that small classification of 'long laborers.' It took nine months to grow that baby and if it takes a while to birth it, so be it. The women thank me when their babies are born. I thank them. I relearn patience from them, time and time again". Jillean

"I have been attending births for twelve years. The most important thing I have learned is each pregnancy, labor, and birth is different. Each woman is different. Each child has its own 'journey' to make, and the mother has hers as well. I used to feel as if I was a guide. I don't think that way anymore. I am really along on the journey, too. It is a privilege to be asked along on another's sacred journey." Marie

"My message is this: Be in love with the whole process and all the people involved. Keep the wonder of it alive inside of you." Karen

"To be the best midwife I can be requires that I must be clear in mind and spirit. I must take care of my physical body–respect it. Anger and hostility interferes with the work I do. I learn, day by day, to relax and flow with birth." Pat

"I became a midwife because I had two cesareans myself. The small town where I live has a 46% c-section rate! With little education, few choices and no support, the women give in to the doctors. I have become an outspoken anti-interventionist. 98% of my mothers, and I take a lot of the so-called high-riskers, have natural deliveries." Carol

"Midwifery is definitely a calling. It's in my cells. It isn't my 'profession' it is part of me. No, it is me. There are no words to tell you the joy, the awesomeness of it all. It is a bit of heaven on this earth." Lianne

Here are some of the things that women who use midwives say about them: They are gentle; they don't injure their clients; they don't use medical interventions; they are so kind to your bottom; they aren't on a power-trip and they don't make you feel guilty or inferior or inadequate; they are patient, they know the meaning of the word "support"; they don't think the doctor's word is God; they are strong in a very loving way; they love babies!; they love women; they know how to listen; they are intuitive; they explain things; they are emotionally accessible; their hands are soft, firm and welcoming; they let me cry and complain; they are warm and compassionate; they are knowledgeable and wise; they know how to build confidence; they're very special, every one of them.

Midwives do not slap a "high-risk" label on a woman as a sentence from which there is no escape. They know steps that can be taken to reduce or eliminate risks. They do not use "gynegadgetry". Midwives often consider a woman a homebirth candidate even when many others would not: her criteria include not only the physical and the physiological, but the nutritional, emotional, psychological, sexual and spiritual, as well. In countless incidences the presence of a midwife has saved women and their babies from unnecessary surgery, unnecessary interventions, episiotomies, and from physical trauma.

Shopping Tips

Purchase a rocking chair for you and your baby. Glider rockers made by Dutailler are an excellent investment and will last for years. A rocking chair is soothing throughout your pregnancy and for those late nights after your baby arrives.

Shopping in your partner's closet can save you time and money. Large T-shirts, baggy pants, an old jogging outfit and even men's underwear with wide waist bands can be very comfortable during the last trimester.

What You Need to Know before You Have Your Baby: Preventing Episiotomy

An episiotomy is a surgical cut through the perineum (the skin and tissue between the vagina and the anus) to widen the birth outlet. A number of doctors are still habitually performing this unnecessary procedure. The practice of episiotomy was initiated in the 1920s by Dr. J.B. Lee who also popularized the "forcep" delivery which he considered the ideal form of birth. Dr. Lee felt that episiotomies were necessary because he believed that a woman's body was not perfectly designed for childbirth. This of course is perfectly untrue.

Today's research on episiotomies, some of which has been conducted by Dr. Michael Klein, Professor of Family Medicine at the University of British Columbia shows that episiotomy can involve a woman's sense of mastery or control over her birth process. Dr. Carolyn DeMarco in her book, *Taking Charge of Your Body* writes, "Episiotomies can be extremely painful – even the most painful part of childbirth" and that "episiotomies are the most common cause of tears." A study by Klein found that women who have episiotomies "resumed sex later, and had more pain during sex and reported less sexual satisfaction, at least in the first three months after birth."

Henci Goer, meta-analysis childbirth researcher and author of *Obstetric Myths Versus Research Realities*, 1995, states, "Routine episiotomy has a ritual function but serves no medical purpose." Goer also reports on the following latest findings: "Episiotomies do not prevent tears into or through the anal sphincter. In fact, deep tears almost never occur in the absence of an episiotomy. Even when properly repaired, tears of the anal sphincter may cause chronic problems with coital pain and gas or fecal incontinence later in life. If a woman does not have an episiotomy, she is likely to have a small tear, but with rare exceptions the tear will be at worse, no worse than a routine episiotomy. Episiotomies do not prevent urinary incontinence or improve sexual satisfaction.

"Episiotomies are not easier to repair than tears. Episiotomies do not heal better than tears. Episiotomies do not prevent birth injuries or fetal brain damage. Episiotomies increase blood loss. As with any other surgical procedure, episiotomies may lead to infection, including fatal infections. Epidurals increase the need for episiotomy. They also increase the probability of instrumental delivery. Instrumental delivery increases both the odds of episiotomy and deep tears. The prone position during delivery increases the need for episiotomy, probably because the perineum is tightly stretched. Some techniques for reducing perineal trauma that have been evaluated and found effective are: prenatal perineal massage, slow delivery of the head, supporting the perineum, keeping the head flexed, delivering the shoulders one at a time, and doing instrumental deliveries without episiotomy."

One of the best midwife's secrets for avoiding an episiotomy is a simple, liberal application of warm oil compresses or warm water compresses applied to your perineum and around your baby's head as it begins to show. A natural tear easily heals on its own. A surgical incision will take twice as long to heal and often leads to deeper and longer tears. The perineum can be compared to a piece of cloth. It is difficult to tear a whole piece of cloth by your hands, but by making cutting a tiny cut into it with scissors the fabric tears easily all the way across. Keeping this area intact should be one of the greatest concerns of your health professionals.

During delivery you will want to stop pushing and pant as your baby's head starts to show and you feel the stretch. Unless there is some medical reason, don't let anyone rush this second stage. Slow and steady at this point will allow your baby's head to be delivered slowly with one shoulder out first and then the other. You need a mirror at this stage to help you to guide your pushing efforts. Your labor assistant will be supporting your perineum by giving gentle counter pressure to your baby's head and your perineum allowing for a safe controlled delivery of the shoulders and chest and will be carefully guiding you throughout this final stage.

What You Need to Know before You Have Your Baby: Induced Birth – Unsafe At Any Speed

Ask your doctor about their personal rate of induced births and under what circumstances they would perform one. Birth is painful enough without the stress effects of a forced or speeded-up labor. If you are planning a normal birth for your baby you may wish for your baby to choose its own birth date. The drugs used to perform an induction are powerful and an induced birth causes both you and your baby to be at great risk. Some doctors feel it is their duty and privilege to remove your baby once you've gone 7 or 10 days past their estimated due date. Most first-time mothers easily go beyond the estimated due date with no harm to the baby or mother whatsoever if they have had a healthy pregnancy. An induction is only indicated if you have experienced any of the following during your pregnancy: heart or kidney disease, pre-eclampsia, diabetes or high blood pressure. An induction should never be done for anyone's convenience. A due date does not have scientific validation due to the wide variation of babies and mothers. There is no way to reliably predict when your baby will be ready to be born. Some babies have easily remained in the womb for up to three and four weeks after the estimated due date. The baby was fine all along; it was the estimation of the date of birth that was wrong. Some doctors are using ultrasounds to estimate due dates. Ultrasounds have not been proven effective in locating the estimated due date. Ultrasounds have also been found to be inaccurate at guessing your baby's weight. The diagnosis that your baby is underweight, small for gestational age, and being told that your placenta is aging can easily frighten any new mother into thinking that her baby needs to be born sooner. When, in fact, the opposite is true. If your baby was under weight you would want to have your baby remain in your womb for as long as possible, as long as you are having a problem-free pregnancy. Unaided, nature shows your body the exact and correct gestation for your baby.

Should your baby at any time in a healthy pregnancy not be growing quickly enough, the simple remedy is to increase your food and liquid intake. You are nourishing your placenta every moment of the day and night and the way to increase the weight of your baby within your womb is to have small meals every two hours, during the day, thus ensuring that nutrition is continually available to you and your baby for as long as it is needed. Current research of placental aging for postmature babies has been shown to have no ill effect on the baby.

A great number of changes must occur within your body in order for a normal, natural birth to happen. Changes are happening within your baby all the way up to the progression of your baby through your birth canal and the last moment when your baby takes the first breath. Normal births are between 38 and 42 weeks and longer. Birth will never be a science, it is designed by nature not man. By allowing your body to reach a natural conclusion to your pregnancy you will have a faster, easier and safer labor and delivery.

Obtain an opinion from other medical support people if your doctor recommends induction for any reason. This medical intervention, called "robbing the cradle," is often done as a convenience for the hospital and staff. Far better to take this extra time to walk, eat, relax and rest for your upcoming position of motherhood. Your baby will appreciate this extra time for growing as well.

Henci Goer in *Obstetrical Myths Versus Research Realities*, 1995, reports the following findings in her meta-analysis of the latest discoveries on inductions: "Median gestational length for first-time mothers exceeds 280 days. First-time mothers have longer pregnancies than second-time mothers. Include one day to gestational length for every day the menstrual cycle normally exceeds 28 days. Healthy fetuses do not lose weight if overdue. Sonographic and clinical weight and date estimates are often wrong. An ultrasound in the first trimester has an error of plus or minus 5 days, increasing to an error rate of plus or minus 8 days in the second trimester and further increasing to an error rate of plus or minus 22 days in the third trimester when estimating due dates. Fetal surveillance tests have high false-positive rates, often showing that there is something wrong when there really isn't. Surveillance tests do not improve outcomes and may increase risk because they lead to intervention. Unilateral breast stimulation safely and effectively ripens the cervix and shortens pregnancy. Routine induction at any stage does not improve perinatal outcome. Inducing increases the risk of fetal distress and cesarean section, especially for first-time mothers."

She also states that "New research shows that in the absence of signs of growth retardation, and in otherwise uncomplicated pregnancies, the safest management of prolonged pregnancy is to await the spontaneous onset of labor. There is a lack of convincing evidence that the overdue fetus is at increased risk of distress or nutritional deprivation. The evidence shows that it is inappropriate to administer prostaglandins for cervical ripening for trivial reasons. The patient must be made aware of all risks of induction."

Risks of the procedure include having to be strapped to an IV or a fetal testing unit or both, causing you to be unable to move about which will slow your baby's descent. You may have accidental or forced rupturing of your membranes leaving you and your baby open to infection and cord prolapse. You will have longer, stronger and more painful contractions causing you to require drugs for pain management. You may have a prolonged labor due to drug usage and an inability to naturally push your baby out due to pain-relieving drugs. Possible oxygen deprivation to your baby can be caused by the extremely long and hard contractions. The next step may be having your baby surgically removed with either an episiotomy with forceps or at the last stage an emergency cesarean section for fetal distress or for failure to progress should your body or baby not be ready to deliver. And so goes the chain of events.

Possible side effects from the induction procedure include post partum hemorrhage, uterine rupture, blood pressure problems, shock and confusion after delivery, prolonged bleeding of six weeks or more, anemia from prolonged blood loss, and possible mental and emotional disturbances, including nightmares and insomnia, and prolonged postnatal depression. Side effects to your baby may include brain damage from oxygen deprivation during labor leading to fetal distress, requiring immediate forced delivery. Should your baby act adversely to the drug or if the induction is not timed correctly your chance of having an emergency cesarean is extremely high, over 50% in some cases.

Your baby may experience cranial hemorrhage and may well become stressed before its first breath. Other risks and side effects of the drugs on the infant are yet to be studied and may include a weakened immune system leading to eczema, asthma, allergies, hives and food intolerances in our babies.

Obstetricians are also using this dangerous drug to speed up labor. The same risks and side effects can occur to both the mother and baby. Studies are now showing that simple nipple stimulation in a stalled labor can have the same effect without any risks or side effects. Once again this is a case where an intervention is used for the convenience of the hospital staff rather than the best interests of the mother and baby.

In *With Child: Birth Through the Ages*, Jenny Carter and Teresa Duriez, 1986, the procedure of induction is put into context with the history of childbirth. "Artificial induction of labor was hardly a new feature of birth intervention; for centuries it has been employed either for motives of self-interest, particularly by 'granny' midwives anxious to get off home, or for medical reasons, such as preventing the mother from having to carry a large fetus. In America in the first decades of this century, it was not uncommon for labor to be hastened so that the delivery of a smaller baby would make the labor easier for the mother. There was no consideration of the possible effect on the child: "Nothing pleased me more in my obstetrical work that to have the baby born a week or two ahead of time . . . Consequently it is not unusual for me to try to 'shake the apple off the tree' ahead of time by using caster oil or quinine, or by starting labor with a rubber bag..."

By the 1940s and 50s, however, it had become common for "fetal indication" to be taken into account when assessing the need for obstetric intervention. That is, doctors began to intervene in the birth process for the sake of the child, even if there were no signs of distress in the mother.

The active management of labor became very much a feature of modern obstetrics following the synthesis of oxytocin and the development of the prostaglandins. Emanuel Friedman in the 1950s presented computations of the average length of time taken in labor by women of various obstetrical histories. If labor did not follow the chart to the satisfaction of the obstetrician a drip was set up to speed up or slow down the process. This process is not as simple as it might sound. One of the disadvantages of using an oxytocin drip to speed up labor is that it tends to increase the strength and frequency of contractions, making pain relief more or less essential. If pethidine or a similar drug is administered to counter the pain, this will in turn slow down the contractions. In order to speed them up again, more oxytocin is given; this in turn causes greater pain and so on.

This particular type of intervention reached its height in Britain in the 1960s and early 70s when induction became not merely a means of protecting mother or fetus, but quite simply a means of achieving the convenient administration and smooth running of the hospital. In 1974, 38% of the births in England and Wales were being induced. And yet 1974 had seen widespread debate about the wisdom of a policy of wholesale induction, and an article in the Lancet in that year concluded that until unequivocal evidence is available, the public is right to question medical practices of doubtful validity that are based on convenience.

Research has now shown that there is a high incidence of fetal distress connected with large doses of oxytocin. An American study found that a slowing down of the fetal heart rate was more common in induced labors, due to a greater intensity of contractions and counter pressure on the fetal head caused by greater resistance of the birth canal. There is no predetermined correct dose of oxytocin.

By the early 1980s the fashion for induction for convenience had almost passed, certainly in Britain. There is no sure way of judging that the time is right for induction and there will inevitably be a proportion of cases in which an error in dating of gestation results in a premature child who may die or suffer irreparable damage in the neonatal period."

In *Take This Book to the Obstetrician with You*, Karla Morales and Charles Inlander, 1991, the authors speak about the controversial nature of inductions. "Hospitals emphasize speed and efficiency. Hospital space is limited and expensive. Every hospital service has its break-even point below which the service loses money, at which it pays for itself, and above which it makes a profit. Obstetrics is no exception. Delivery suites must reflect a high turnover rate to pay the mortgage on the first of the month and staff salaries every other Friday. From an economic point of view, hospitals cannot afford to allow women to labor at their own natural, unhurried pace.

The usual interventions employed are amniotomy to induce labor and intravenous administration of Pitocin or vaginal application of Prostin to stimulate labor. What's the problem with artificial augmentation of labor? Just ask any woman who has been given Pitocin, the common synthetic version of the hormone oxytocin. Many, if not most, will report longer and stronger contractions and shorter intervals between contractions than they experience in unstimulated labor. Thus, the stage is set for yet another intervention, in this case painkilling drugs for the relief of contractions of overwhelming intensity. As for possible adverse effects of elective stimulation of labor on the fetus, various reports relate how the strength and rapidity of contractions can decrease the ability of the fetus to restore its supply of oxygen between contractions. So the door swings open to yet another intervention, perhaps forceps delivery or a cesarean section. Ask your doctor about his percentage of induced labors. Doctors who perform inductions for medical indications only induce less than

10 percent – some less than 5 percent."

If you feel your induction was for a vague or clinically unsubstantiated reason and would like to voice your objection to being subjected to the latest weapon in the arsenal of birth medical interventions, write to your hospital. Some hospital policies and procedures have been changed with as few as a dozen letters voicing complaint of certain procedures. Send the original letter to the College of Physicians and Surgeons listed in the white pages of your telephone directory. There is no time limit on sending your letter and a lawyer is not necessary to have your concern heard. Include the name of your doctor, hospital name and address, reasons for induction given by your doctor and what happened to you and your baby as a result of this medical intervention. Some babies have a delayed reaction that may show up in excessive newborn crying, food intolerances, sensitivities and allergies, especially dairy intolerances, hives, persistent eczema and asthma in the infant. One of the greatest risks to the mother beyond hemorrhage is prolonged and severe postnatal depression. Your letter will make a difference for the others who come after you and will help doctors understand why we object to this painful, dangerous and increasingly common birth intervention.

6

Sixth Month

Drink extra water. Keep a glass beside you at your desk and sip on it during the day. Remember you are flushing the waste of two people now. Do not hold your urine in when you need to go as this can cause bladder and kidney infections. Your bladder holds a smaller amount now, so you must adjust for that by urinating more frequently.

Do not lie flat on your back. Always lie on your side, preferably your left side, to avoid constricting your blood flow and oxygen to your baby. This includes during your prenatal visits, sleeping, and of course during your labor and delivery.

Natural Remedies for Heartburn

If you find yourself a victim of heartburn, before reaching for the Tums or Maalox, look to your diet. Eat plenty of raw food with each meal. Plan to eat only raw fruits and vegetable for one day to re-establish your digestive enzymes to break the cycle of heartburn. Make sure each meal contains raw fruits or vegetables. You can also buy digestive enzymes at the health food store and take them with every meal.

Eat your largest meal earlier in the day. Snack on fruit or vegetables in the early evening. Celery is a great antidote if heartburn strikes during the evening when you are out. Make sure to chew the fruit or vegetables well to release the enzymes.

When sleeping, you may want to arrange your pillows so that you are in a semi-reclining position.

Avoid foods that are fatty or greasy. Foods that are too acid or too spicy may also bother you. Stay away from carbonated drinks, processed meats and junk foods.

Avoid using antacids that contain aluminum or bicarbonate of soda. These can interfere with absorption of certain nutrients, upset your acid base balance and possibly harm your baby.

Calcium in the form of pills, powder or liquid is a natural antacid and can be used in doses of up to 1,200 mg per day. Magnesium should always be taken with calcium at about half the dosage of the calcium.

One teaspoon of slippery elm bark powder which is found in health food stores mixed with honey or hot water neutralizes stomach acidity and soothes the stomach.

When you travel, you can carry raw almonds and chew on them slowly to help relieve heartburn.

Natural Remedies for Muscle Cramping

Keep pillows under your knees or feet to reduce cramping while you are sleeping. If you get a bad cramp during the night flex your toes and feet forward while still lying down to stretch those muscles. Rotate your ankles. If the cramp is really strong, stand up and put your weight on it. Drinking more water during the day will help to ease evening leg cramps. Calcium tablets have also been found to help relieve cramping.

Natural Remedies for Food Cravings

If you are experiencing salt and sweet cravings you have a nutritional deficiency known as Pica. If you are experiencing intense cravings add a liquid mineral supplement to your diet. In horses and milk cows this is called cribbing. When this happens to an animal you add minerals to their diet.

Prenatal Classes

Start looking for an independent childbirth instructor now. Some hospital supported prenatal classes promote the various medical interventions offered at their hospital. The best value for your money is an independent instructor who will talk to you about avoiding unnecessary medical interventions, natural pain relief methods, and the emotional and spiritual aspects of birth. The more knowledge you acquire about the birth process the faster and easier your labor and delivery will be. Take a partner, if you have one, if not go alone.

Many prenatal courses are available over a weekend or a couple of weekdays. Ask for referrals from your health team to find the best class. Each class will have its own ideas or philosophies about the birth process, interview the instructors to see if their ideas match yours. Read your birth plan over the telephone to make sure they have experience in the birth you want for your baby. Look in the Childbirth Resource Directory located in this guide for referrals on independent childbirth educators in your city.

Home Work

If at this point you are feeling large and awkward and wondering how you are going to get your house cleaned, set up a plan for yourself. It may just seem like too much of an effort all at once and it is. Try doing one or two things each day. For example, dust on Monday, wash sheets and towels on Tuesday, have someone else vacuum on Wednesday, sweep and mop the floor on Thursday, do the bathrooms on Friday, clean the kitchen on Saturday, and do laundry on Sunday! Keeping things as tidy as possible and 'put away' each day also helps. Your home may not be all clean all at the same time, but each job gets done in turn. Hire someone to mow your lawn or shovel your sidewalk. You will find that once your baby arrives, the same principles apply.

Keep your good humor! Things can and will go wrong. Realize that simple tasks may become difficult either because of your increasing size or because of your preoccupation. You will forget things and you may be unable to manage some tasks that were part of your everyday routine. So, when you burn supper or forget to return a phone call or can't reach that top shelf in the kitchen cabinets, remember these are short-term problems that you can shrug off.

What You Need to Know before You Have Your Baby: Preventing Cesarean Birth

Excerpted from Take This Book to the Obstetrician with You, *Karla Morales and Charles B. Inlander, 1991*

Of all the issues you face as you prepare for childbirth, cesarean section is the most controversial: the hands-down winner if you are looking for the topic that raises the most eyebrows in a group of childbirth educators, sets the majority of tongues and chins wagging in a meeting of obstetricians, and appears regularly in medical journals, popular magazines, and newspapers nationwide. Ralph Nader's Public Citizen Health Research Group says that it is the number one "unnecessary surgery" in the United States. Health policy analysts, renegade voices within the medical profession, and consumer groups call it a national epidemic. And just about every critic dubs it the ultimate medical intervention in childbirth.

Today, one of four pregnant women in the United States and one in twenty pregnant women in Canada will give birth by cesarean section – a rate higher than any other country in the world, according to the National Center for Health Statistics. Britain considers its 11% cesarean rate a crisis. At one time, c-section was considered a last resort, an emergency lifesaving event for mother and baby. "A less than 5% rate for a practitioner was a hallmark of good obstetric practice," reports the *Journal of the American Medical Association* 1989 editorial. In 1970, the rate of cesarean births in this country stood at just 5.5% of all live births. But between 1970 and 1987 the rate skyrocketed to its present level – without a corresponding drop in the infant or maternal mortality rate.

Traditionally, c-section has been considered medically necessary and safer than vaginal birth in a number of high-risk situations, including multiple birth, delivery of a large infant, delivery involving a woman with a serious condition or health problem such as infection, separation of the placenta from the uterine wall, or where the placenta extends over the opening of the cervix, prolapse of the umbilical cord and breech birth.

Mortimer Rosen, MD, chairman of Columbia University medical school's department of obstetrics and gynecology, has written one of the definitive books on this topic. *In The Cesarean Myth*, 1989, he sets forth and subsequently refutes three key myths concerning cesareans:

1. A belief that they are safe. On the contrary, he says, as a form of major surgery, the emergency c-section poses a 400 percent higher risk of death to the mother than does vaginal birth, and elective cesarean a 200 percent higher risk. Not only is the recovery period longer and more difficult but certain complications are nearly impossible to avoid: pain, infection, the aftereffects associated with anesthesia, such as migraines, as well as bleeding, sometimes excessive enough to require a transfusion.

2. A belief that they are absolutely necessary in a broad range of situations. Along with others, Rosen says that the need for a c-section should be evaluated on a case-by-case basis because only a few broadly defined conditions or predicaments warrant the intervention, such as certain breech births and situation in which the placenta is attached in the wrong place. Clearly that cautionary approach is not in force in medical practice today. Instead, when doctors come across any uncertainty in the progress of labor or anything less than perfectly normal, many of them call for the operating room and the knife. With so many doctors racing to the operating room and hustling women into surgery, a lot of women are having cesareans even though the diagnosis may be vague or clinically unsubstantiated.

3. A belief that they produce healthier, "better" babies. Rosen echoes many other experts in the field who find no substantive evidence that c-sections are better for babies than vaginal deliveries. The recent dramatic rise in cesareans, he says, has not reduced overall infant mortality rates or produced a generation of healthier babies. The United States has one of the highest rates of infant mortality in the world according to the Centers for Disease Control calculations. And as a major surgery, a cesarean section poses risks not only for the mother but also for the baby, including risk of iatrogenic, doctor caused, conditions including respiratory distress and carry-over effects from the drugs and anesthetics given the mother and infant.

Other less indulgent critics of cesareans who have looked deeper into the heart of the beast say that myths do not tell the whole story, that there are rampant nonmedical motivations at work here. Herbert H. Keyser, MD in his book *Women under the Knife: A Gynecologist's Report on Hazardous Medicine* 1984, calls the following "the dark side" of the increase in cesareans:

The Profit Motive: Cesareans are more lucrative than normal vaginal deliveries. The doctor's fee is higher, the hospital stay is longer – more than twice as long as vaginal deliveries, says a *Journal of the American Medical Association* 1990 article, with an average stay somewhere around four to five days, assuming no complications. A cost survey by Modern Healthcare 1990 shows $5,133 as the average hospital charge, and $2,053 the average physician charge, and so a cesarean birth typically costs $7,186. This stacks up against $2,111, the average cost of a one-day stay in a birthing center for a normal delivery, a figure that includes professional fees. As for a midwife assisted vaginal delivery, her average charge is $994.

The Convenience Factor: A typical scenario finds the obstetrician sitting around the hospital doctors' lounge or nurses' station waiting for a woman's labor to run its course so that the doctor can be there for her in the minutes before birth. But what if her labor, as many other women's before her, takes longer than scheduled? If it is the beginning of the day, the doctor has patients to see during office hours, and at the end of the day, well, there are other commitments, possibly even a golf game. Even if the woman desires to labor longer, why wait to see whether there truly is a problem? Not only does inactivity waste the doctor's time, but it does not pay very well either. Given such economics, is it not easier for the doctor to consider possible fetal distress or possible dystocia and opt for a c-section? Keyser says that except for previously scheduled cesarean sections which are usually done in the early morning, by far the greatest number are done immediately after office hours.

A Lack of Education and Training: Obstetrical training emphasizes high-risk care and the extensive use of technology in labor and delivery. Doctors today receive very little training and experience in normal deliveries with one in four births a cesarean. The skills, such as those required to turn around breech babies for vaginal deliveries, just are not there. A study of more than six thousand deliveries at a New York City hospital reported in the July 1989 *American Journal of Obstetrics and Gynecology*, found some correlation between physician characteristics and the cesarean rate: namely, that older, more experienced doctors perform significantly fewer cesarean sections for difficult labor.

Entrenched Practice Patterns: How else to explain the variation in cesarean rates from practitioner to practitioner, hospital to hospital, and region to region? Practice habits, peer pressure, and other nonmedical factors seem to play a large role. Many doctors are reluctant to try tactics, for example, that were used successfully by midwives for centuries to help delivering women overcome problems in labor: changes in birth position, change in environment, walking, warm shower or bath, and breast and nipple stimulation.

If you've had a previous cesarean birth, locate a doctor or midwife that will encourage you to have a normal vaginal birth. Contact the Vaginal Birth After Cesarean Group (VBAC) in your area for excellent information and health teams to support you all the way. VBAC groups are listed in the Childbirth Resource Directory in this guide. The July 1991 report of the Ontario Government's Cesarean Birth planning committee estimates that more that 65% out of 11,000 repeat cesareans could have been prevented. Research in this field is now showing that many first cesareans could also have been avoided given fewer medical interventions in labor and personalized labor support for the mother and father.

Vaginal Birth After Cesarean

Excerpted from Silent Knife: Cesarean Prevention and Vaginal Birth After Cesarean, *Nancy Wainer Cohen and Lois J. Estner, 1983*

Vaginal birth after cesarean is not only safe but generally safer than its alternative. In spite of the research, evidence and documentation that appear on this subject, most obstetricians in this country continue to perform repeat cesareans simply because a woman has been previously sectioned. There is always an excuse, it seems, why a woman cannot be a candidate for vaginal birth after cesarean or a vaginal birth in the first place. We know that most women who have had a cesarean are capable of delivering vaginally. This includes women with a diagnosis of cephalo-pelvic disproportion, (CPD), prolonged labor or failure to progress, (FTP), or more than one previous cesarean. We have worked with women who have had vaginal births after cesarean, VBAC breech births, VBAC twins, and many other VBAC special circumstances.

We know that women who want to birth vaginally after a cesarean are not crazy, selfish or insane. We know that many cesarean women are bitter and sorrowful. There is great understanding for a man who is unable to get an erection or ejaculate; most people understand that this is a part of his total identity as a male. There is support for feelings of inadequacy, frustration, failure, sadness and guilt. But there is very little understanding for cesarean women who have feelings of disappointment, sadness, failure, and frustration at not being able to complete the normal womanly physiological process of giving birth. For many women, becoming pregnant and giving birth are integrally and intricately linked with feelings of self-worth and identity. It is any wonder that so many women in our culture are grieving? To want to give birth in a way that unites us with other women, to all women. To want to experience each of the cycles of our life is not insane. It is normal. We must take a careful look at our obstetrical practices, whether or not that scrutiny upsets or threatens the medical establishment.

What You Need to Know before You Have Your Baby: Cesarean Awareness: The Politics of Birth

Excerpted from Open Season – A Survival Guide for Natural Childbirth and Vaginal Birth After Cesarean in the 90's *Nancy Wainer Cohen, 1991*

The rate of prenatal testing, drugs, IVs, monitoring equipment, induction agents, forceps, and vacuum extractions, for example, has increased in the past ten years, despite the vast amount of information cautioning against them and despite the high percentage of couples in this country who go through "prepared-childbirth" classes. This is a joke. Couples taught in hospitals are rarely prepared to have their babies, rather, they are prepared for induced labors and pain killers, for having their water broken, and for episiotomies, all of which are invasive, unnecessary, and complicate the birth process. These couples are alternately courted, humored, intimidated, and patronized. They're lied to. Not surprisingly, cesarean sections among hospital trained couples also continue to increase, turning the illness into a plague. Babies are drugged out, forced out, pulled, pushed, sucked, or sliced out of their mothers' "prepared" bodies, and both parties are left to "recover" from the experience.

If childbirth classes really worked, more women would be having babies without interference. More women would recognize the complete naturalness of birth and would remain at home, delivering their infants with feelings of confidence and trust.   More and more midwives would be demanded. If childbirth classes worked, birth paraphernalia would be used less and less rather than more and more. If the classes worked, if they truly prepared women to deliver their babies, then women would be delivering them. Instead, women are delivered of their infants through the wonders of medical technology, by the wielders of those technologies. For all the good that hospital childbirth classes may have set out to do, few have done much, and little has changed. Thousands of naive pregnant couples, listen to unqualified childbirth educators teaching nothing more than a glorified biology lesson, dishing out misleading and unenlightening information, and who thus deliver their couples into the waiting hands of equally unqualified members of the obstetrical establishment. Few American women survive prepared childbirth without suffering indignities that leave them scarred for years to come.

It is not only childbirth educators that bear responsibility. Medical schools and nursing schools are also at fault. Ginny Cassidy-Brinn, co-author of *Woman-Centered Pregnancy and Birth,* remarks that she has become thoroughly convinced that her nursing instructors were abysmally ignorant about normal childbirth. "Most students finish their obstetrical rotations no longer believing in the process of birth. In fact, few have ever even seen a purebirth. I was not surprised, but nonetheless appalled, to learn that not one of the nursing students to whom I spoke had seen a natural birth. Two thought they had, but when I reminded them that enemas, IVs, and episiotomies do not constitute a natural birth, they realized that natural births did not take place in their institutions. Most were horrified or repulsed by their obstetrical rotation and were extremely fearful of giving birth themselves". Obstetrical students rarely understand or experience the broad variations that may occur in normal birth. They are severely limited by what they are taught is within safe boundaries. Their boundaries become our barbed-wire fences, leaving each of us little freedom to do our own births in our own way. Few medically trained students know what roles herbs, chiropractic care, acupuncture, homeopathy, or a change in beliefs, for example, can play in helping a woman have her baby.

Hospital administrations are equally responsible. It is time that physicians be required to make their statistics public. A woman should be able to know the number of births a particular care provider has attended and of these the number of cesareans performed. In addition, she should be able to ascertain how many of the women were monitored, had IVs, drugs, forceps, vacuum extractions and episiotomies.

Politicians, legislators, and insurance companies are responsible. Cesarean section remains an enormous political, legal, and economic football. Many decisions that affect mother, baby, family are made perhaps unconsciously for personal, institutional, and bureaucratic gain.

The media are responsible. I am constantly amazed at the number of people quoted as experts in the field of obstetrics who have never been pregnant, never felt a contraction, never had a baby; many of them don't even have a vagina! Women all over the country who are truly the experts are frequently not considered a reliable or knowledgeable source of information.

Television is of little help. Soap operas haven't changed since Lois and I first reported to you, and they continue to give us erroneous insights into present cultural attitudes about birth. On Friday afternoon, viewers are still left hanging by a thread. Will the emergency cesarean save her baby? The natural births that have been shown in the last few years have been good for nothing more than a belly laugh. Mother holding her breath turning beet red. Father, dressed in green, looking like part of the anesthesiology staff, secretly wishing someone would put him out. Nurse, instructing Mother to PUUUUUSH with all her might. Everyone draped, instruments readied, doctor in control. These scenes bear no resemblance to what normal birth is and no understanding of what childbirth can or should be.

Of course in the end we are all responsible. Childbirth educator and author Cathy Romeo comments, "Instead of encouraging women to feel capable and powerful during the birth experience, most people contribute to the woman feeling helpless and frightened. If a man were giving birth, would we say, "Don't worry about a thing, dear, everything will be taken care of." No, we'd say, "Go get 'em, tiger!!!!"

In my opinion, I'm certain that at least 97 percent of cesarean sections are preventable and therefore unnecessary. Women and babies are far more hurt than helped by cesarean section. Maternal deaths are four times greater after cesarean section and the complications for babies are astronomical. Dr. Michele Odent has often said that anyone with two hands and a few instruments can do a cesarean section, it frequently requires great intelligence not to do it.

Women have been told that cesareans are "the best route" for the baby and that women should opt for cesarean. Dr. Sidney Wolfe, head of the Public Citizen Health Research Group, says that cesareans are the number one unnecessary surgery in this country and that "Mothers are not being adequately informed of the risks involved to themselves and their babies."

Patricia Newell of the Cesarean Prevention Movement says that cesarean section may contribute to secondary infertility and that this may be one of the least recognized and most emotionally devastating long-term aftereffects of cesarean section. Newell reports that a cesarean heightens the chance of one-child infertility. Beth Shearer, co-director of C/Sec, has noted that a significant number of women who have had cesareans have endometriosis, and up to 50% of women found to have scarring do not become pregnant again.

Even breech preemies do far better vaginally delivered than surgically removed. This makes so much sense when you remember that even full-term cesarean babies have much more difficulty breathing. They have a greatly increased incidence of hyaline membrane disease, immature lungs. Labor helps to ready the infant for survival outside the mother's body; it matures the lungs. Tiny babies, so often delivered by c-section in this country do better when they can experience labor and be stimulated to breathe by the cyclical rhythms of the contractions and by the natural passage through their mother's bodies into the world.

What about big breech babies? The only intervention is to insist that the woman be in a supported squatting position. Many women have delivered large breech babies – they either remained at home or came into the hospital pushing. There are positions and exercises for turning breech babies, and many of them work. Doctors often panic because they don't have the slightest notion how to attend a breech birth; rather than admit it, they frighten you into a cesarean for which they have plenty of experience. Doctors could learn a great deal about breech deliveries from homebirth midwives. Some women have turned their babies by simply talking to them or by writing a letter to them. Some have used acupuncture points, acupressure points, reflexology, healing touch, homeopathic remedies, and herbs. One woman spent a few days swimming in a pool – she played like a child in the water, doing gentle turns and slow somersaults – and the baby turned. Other women have done absolutely nothing at all, and their babies have turned.

It's hard to imagine what it would be like to be forced into a c-section. Yet, in a sense we are all forced: we wouldn't allow ourselves to be cut open unless we believed it was necessary or unless our internal fear prevented us from birthing normally. We are all forced to comply – it is a form of forced consent. Many people think that a woman who undergoes a cesarean section recovers and gets on with her life. Sadly, this is not always the case. The physical and psychological repercussions of cesarean sections are numerous and grim. The women who have written me, letters I have quoted throughout this book, were not trying to scare anyone when they wrote to me. They themselves were scared and they were simply telling their story. Judy Herzffeld in *Sense and Sensibility* says that if the American pregnant woman could only learn a few words, she'd be in good shape, such as: "stop, wait, slow, take it off, take it away, go away, be quiet, when I'm ready, when it's time."

The other diagnoses given to mothers to convince them to have cesarean sections are:

Fetal Distress – Not a good enough reason. Usually reported by faulty mechanical heart measuring. Insist on a manual device, like a fetoscope or stethoscope to monitor your baby's progress. Baby Too Large – Not a good enough reason. No one and no machine can yet predict the exact weight of a baby in the womb. Pelvis Too Small – Not a good enough reason. As above, no one is able to predict accurate pelvis size or accurate weight of baby. Failure to Progress – Not a good enough reason. Take a walk instead. Or better yet, have your health team take a walk. If you feel that your labor has stalled, move, walk, climb stairs, squat, kneel, lean over something or someone, belly dance, tap dance, have a shower, or a bath in a darkened room, turn up or turn down the lights, turn up or turn down the music, clear everyone out of the room or invite new people in, talk to a good friend who is far away, open the windows and breathe fresh air. Your movement and activity will greatly assist you and your baby at this time, your body will naturally and instinctively do the work.

Here are some letters from women who refused a second cesarean section:

Cathy: For three years I maintained my cesarean was unnecessary and six months ago I proved it! My cesarean was for cpd-ftp (small pelvis/large baby and failure to progress). It turned out he was actually a 7 pound boy with a 13 1/2 inch head. My purebirth son was 9 1/2 pounds with a 15 inch head. I left the first group of doctors I had because they refused to allow me to labor, although they did promise me a meaningful cesarean. I switched to a doctor who said he supports VBACs. When I was nine months pregnant, he changed his mind. I changed doctors again. The hospital where I work as an aide won't tell you the truth, but they do almost 70% cesareans.

Claudia: We did it! A VBAC after two cesareans! Trying to negotiate with eight doctors in the area took too much energy. After lots of discussion, our midwife friend agreed to be at home with us. During labor, I tried to forget everything I knew about birth and follow my instincts. Two days of labor and Logan was born. Never once did I lose confidence!

Janine: I was sectioned at age sixteen by an impatient older doctor who admitted me in my warm-up phase of labor. He sent me for x-rays and cut me for a slightly flattened sacrum – all other measurements normal. The second was a repeat cesarean with a different incision and now I had a T. I had about seven hours of early labor and six hours of active. I pushed for about 90 minutes and the placenta came out an hour later. At one point, my midwife had a "heart to heart" talk with me. She said I had to want it to get stronger. She told me she would hold my hand and lead me to the next phase, and to not be afraid. She moaned with me and then asked me to change my moan to a whisper and say yes. Ten minutes later I said "I've got to push!" Incidentally, my mother was at the birth. She was a tower of strength, having undergone an unnecessary section with her third child.

Chris: I took heart tones on my own. When I was completely dilated, my water broke. There was a moderate amount of meconium. After a number of hours, I said to myself, "No one else can do this for me. I might as well get to it." And so I did.

Lisa: I did it! It's a boy! Two years of hard work paid off in a wonderful birth experience for us. I can hardly believe it! I have healed my cesarean scar. I am woman! Things slowed down a few times but no one got concerned. I just got in the shower and stayed there until I felt a strong desire to push. It took me a little while to find out how to best direct my energy toward effective pushing. His head circumference was nearly an inch bigger than his brother's who was born by section for cpd. I had no episiotomy and no tearing, thanks to perineal massage during late pregnancy, kegel exercises, more massage during crowning, and a slow easy delivery assisted by my midwife. There was some fetal distress just before the birth, but a change in position helped that. The cord was looped around his head twice, but Shelly slipped it over his head and left it uncut.

Lynne: My cesarean was done for cpd. What a laugh. This baby, born at home, was what they called a compound presentation. His hand was up next to the side of his head and just as the head was showing we saw a hand and the arm up there, too. My son still sleeps with his arm near his head.

Loretta: My doctor remarked that waiting for our baby was like having three coronaries. He stayed at the hospital all night – he slept in the doctors' lounge. He'd never attended a woman with one cesarean before, let alone me with two. The nurse told me to be a good girl and leave the fetal monitor belts on. I informed her that good little girls end up with c-sections, that women get pregnant and have babies, not girls.

Rosie: I was able to achieve my fantasy about childbirth at home with a midwife. Amazingly, I labored for only two hours, it began when I put my first two down for a nap and Sophie was born when they woke up! It was a real family event. The boys made a birthday cake and we had balloons and flowers delivered to the house. An hour after she was born, we celebrated her very first birthday. What I liked best was nothing in our normal daily routine was changed. The boys went to bed their usual time that night. As a result, the boys accepted her arrival very matter of factly, naturally, and without jealousy. What a difference from my cesareans.

Jon: I called you a few months ago. My wife has a classical scar from a cesarean section. Although we have never met, I knew you would be happy to know the result, a beautiful homebirth with a midwife. Her labor was 57 hours and she pushed for an additional three. Our baby was 9 lbs 4 ounces.

Jean: It only took four hours from start to finish, and five minutes later I felt marvelous! That's how birth should be, isn't it? A 10 pound VBAC son.

Adrean: An update! We just had our second home VBAC after four days with broken membranes. Midwives are so patient! Automatic labor didn't click in until the fourth day, lasted for about 45 minutes, and then, seven minutes of hard, overwhelming pushing and it was all over! She arrived with her little arm right alongside her head. The birth ended up quite a party, the midwives who were taking turns here all stayed, all four of our other kids were there, and my dear friend was camerawoman! This birth confirmed how different each labor and delivery is even in the same woman and to keep it in the confines of a chart or graph is so ludicrous!

Claire: My pushing phase was eight hours. I had read about a VBAC woman who pushed for twelve. I was hoping not to win the record, but knowing that there is wide variation to all phases of labor helped me. I am so proud.

Gretta: I called you when I was four weeks overdue. I went into labor four days later, and had a perfect baby and a great birth. Quick, relatively easy. Home in eight hours.

Karen: I spent the better part of this pregnancy working to get into the birthing room. I had two previous sections and a T incision. They hooked me up to a malfunctioning fetal monitor and told me they couldn't get the baby's heartbeat. My professional labor support had brought her trusty fetoscope and the heartbeat was strong and steady throughout.

Michalene: The magic of this experience will last forever. I realize that I set myself up to win. It has changed me and us. I have given birth. I am humbled. Not just by the birth but by the overwhelming support everyone has given me. With no strings, and with complete total devotion. This is the most exciting, exhilarating, strongest experience of my life.

It is your responsibility to yourself and your baby to get second and third opinions from other professionals who are experienced in normal birth should there ever be any discussion of a cesarean section surgery. If you need to pay for these other opinions on your own you should do so. Call the nearest Childbirth Association, discuss your situation and you will be immediately connected with a specialist in your area.

As we begin to take our births back we are also creating a new language to go with the experience of purebirth:

Contractions become Babyhugs

Amniotic Fluid becomes a Cradlebasket

Second stage becomes Babytime

Cesarean birth is "Open Uterine Surgery" or even "Ouch" open uterine cutting at the hospital

Dilation becomes Opening, Unfolding, Expanding

Mucus plug becomes Babygel

Labor sounds become Birth Music.

Today you can get tested for everything from A to Z. The choices you make may depend in large part on the system you choose, medical or nonmedical, on the paradigm you adopt and on the beliefs you carry in your heart about birth. The choices you make for yourself during your pregnancy will influence those you make during your labor. If you believe that birth is a natural process, which it is, you will see that the majority of modern day medical interventions are just that. An intervention into what should be a normal, natural occurrence in a woman's body.

We must challenge our beliefs about birth continually. Here are some of my basic beliefs about birth:

- Birth is a normal physiological process that does not require tools, tubes, chemicals, drugs, machines or doctors.
- Women and babies are designed to experience childbirth; they are designed to come through the experience safely and unharmed.
- The pain of childbirth is healthy, normal, appropriate pain.
- The spiritual, emotional, psychological and sexual environments in which a woman births are as important as other considerations, such as the size of her pelvis or the size of the baby, as a matter of fact, more important.
- The attitude in our country that doctors deliver babies rather than the belief that women give birth perpetuates the high rate of unnatural births.
- Political and economic incentives also perpetuate the problem.
- Any intervention into the birth process can, and most likely will, confuse the body and upset the process. This is true whether the interference is medical, physiological, or emotional.

Birth is a significant life experience. Its effects are long lasting. It must be an experience which honors women, babies, families, and society at large. Women are capable, strong human beings who are fully able to meet the challenges of giving birth, especially if they have information and support, but even without these. There are very few reasons for intervention, and very few reasons for a cesarean section. These should be reserved for the rare occasions when Mother Nature needs a bit of assistance, not as routine procedures to get the baby out. If a woman with a previous cesarean does not feel that her body is healed, she will not allow a subsequent labor to become strong enough to birth the baby. No woman will continue to labor if she believes that the labor will harm her or her baby. For a woman to feel physically healed, emotional healing is usually necessary. If the men or women who attend women at birth have upset, unfinished business, or fear about birth, or if their belief systems are not conducive to normal birthing, these thoughts may affect the birthing woman. We must all work to heal on physiological and spiritual levels about birth. Good nutrition is essential for pregnancy and birth. Most doctors know beans about the vital role that nutrition plays and often harm women with their diets and recommendations.

Maternal well-being, the healthy integration of the birth experience, is of paramount importance. It is the woman's responsibility to birth her baby and to make the decisions leading to this time in her life. It is not the doctor's or the institution's or the midwife's decision. Women get to choose who and how many people they want at birth. They get to kick out anybody they don't want or like. The caring fathers of the soon to be born babies are extremely vulnerable in the hospital setting. They often become the doctor's cohort, with the woman and baby the pawns. Fathers are birthing too and together with the mother they deserve and need support and reassurance as well. Each of us is either an advocate for birth or for the system. At this point in time, the two are mutually exclusive. We cannot be both. The system is not an advocate for women or babies or birth. If you don't want an episiotomy, or a forceps delivery, or a cesarean section, you simply make certain that when you are in labor you have chosen a place where these procedures are unable to be performed. It is as simple as that.

7

Seventh Month

This is a good time to preview the section in this book on newborn care. Visualize what you will do with your baby on your first day together. More women are using Kangaroo Care on the first day, letting baby sleep or nap on your chest with skin to skin contact after feeding to help maintain the close connection your baby felt to you in your womb. It is a wonderful way to soothe both mother and baby in the first days together. Kangaroo care by both partners creates deeper bonding and attachment with your baby. The scent of your baby actually releases certain hormones to help both partners bond more closely with the baby. This is why we can't resist kissing baby's sweet cheeks. Their scent is truly irresistible.

To relieve pressure on your body while sleeping add a second pillow to prop you up as you sleep. This can help you to breathe easier and can help relieve heartburn. Sleeping with a pillow tucked slightly under your belly can also relieve any muscle straining you may be feeling. Body pillows give great support to your expanding body and belly. They are available at most department stores like the Bay, Sears, Eatons, Walmart and Zellers.

Fill small plastic bottles with one third juice and two thirds water and store in your freezer. Take a frozen bottle with you for the car or at work for a cool refreshing drink.

Stock up on sodium-free club soda. Soda has no calories and is great for quenching your thirst. Keep a stock in your car and at work.

Purchase good slippers with some elastic support. Try Isotoner slippers for a great fit.

Increase your outdoor activities. Animals give birth faster and easier when they are let free once a day rather than being penned up. A rancher did an independent study by putting half his pregnant cattle within the corral day and night, the other half were led to a feeding area a distance away every evening. Twice as many complications arose in the cows that had been penned up. Giving birth is a tremendous physical challenge to your body and the stronger you become physically, the easier the challenge.

Walking will ease lower back pain and is a great way to unwind from the day. If you have back pain you may want to walk on a treadmill at a gym or walk on grass. Shopping malls have tile placed upon concrete which can create additional pressure on your back and legs. You will also find that walking strengthens muscles you will be using during your labor and delivery. Stronger legs allow you to maintain an assisted squatting position for a longer period of time. A squatting position is one of the best and most natural positions for birth making for an easier delivery for both mother and baby.

Can't sleep near the end of your pregnancy? Get up and do something useful or relaxing. Nature is getting you ready for the time when you will have to get up in the middle of the night, so learn to use the time for your benefit. There may be many nights when your baby is a few months old and she is awake at 2:00 a.m. for one or two hours. You can prepare yourself for this by learning how to amuse yourself during these times. After your baby is fed and changed, she may still want to play for awhile or just be awake. You can sit with her and read a book or get a snack or whatever. Some mothers videotape their favorite daytime shows for late night-viewing during these times.

Kegels

Kegels reduce urinary incontinence, help relieve and reduce hemorrhoids, help you to create a faster and easier delivery and will get you ready and toned again to resume a good sex life. To locate your muscle and do the Kegel exercises; when urinating start and stop the flow of urine, this will isolate the target muscle area which is the PC muscle. Tighten these muscles and hold to the count of ten, then release and tighten again. Latest research shows that holding your PC muscles for a long rather than a short period of time will condition these muscles more quickly. Count to ten and slowly release for the greatest effect in the shortest amount of time. To keep your PC muscle toned it is important to practice Kegel exercises on a daily basis, both before and after the birth. Do sets of ten or twenty throughout the day.

Other variations include; Slow Kegels: tighten the PC muscle as if to stop the urine. Hold for a slow count of three, and then relax. Repeat ten times. Quick Kegels: Tighten and relax the PC muscle as quickly as you can, five times. Relax and repeat ten times. Pull in-Push Out Kegels: Pull up the entire pelvic floor as though trying to suck water into the vagina. Then push out or bear down as if trying to push imaginary water out. This exercise uses the stomach abdominal muscles as well as the PC muscle. Do this four or five times in a row. Repeat ten times.

Sex after Childbirth

Pregnancy, labor and delivery are taxing on a woman's body. How the mother cares for herself and is cared for, after the baby comes, depends on the nature of the delivery and whether there have been any complications. It is important to get up and around as soon as possible after childbirth for the healing of your body. Be guided by your own body. Activities such as work, sex, housework, and exercise should be resumed when you feel ready. In Western culture, people have demanding schedules and are used to instant results. It is therefore important for a woman to be aware of the stress her body has endured and the recovery it must make. Sleep deprivation, breastfeeding, and caring for your infant and yourself make extra demands on your body. Pacing yourself and taking slow steps are key in maintaining normal activities and optimum health. Good nutrition while breastfeeding remains as important now as during pregnancy. Eating a varied diet with plenty of whole foods and fluids still applies. Aggressive dieting during this time of healing and nurturing is detrimental to the health of both mother and baby.

A woman must determine for herself when she is ready to resume intercourse. Probably the most important thing to feed a healthy sex life is a healthy relationship. Parents are often taught that children come first. But if a marriage or relationship is not attended to, there is no family. Partners should get out by themselves on a regular basis and find ways to attend to each other emotionally and not just sexually. In this way you will reconnect with the relationship you had before your first baby.

Setting aside ten or fifteen minutes per day for discussing the events of the day is a pleasant way for partners to reconnect. Sleep is a powerful aphrodisiac and can contribute to both partners enjoyment of sex when you set the alarm for the middle of the night. Hiring a baby-sitter away from home in the middle of the day when both partners are more rested can also help you to resume sexual activity and intimacy. Doing Kegel exercises throughout your pregnancy and after birth will quickly recondition your body. Using extra lubricant during lovemaking at this time can also make sexual activity more enjoyable.

Fear of another pregnancy often decreases a woman's sexual desires after childbirth. Plan ahead for your birth control method. While breastfeeding appears to suppress ovulation somewhat and helps in the spacing of children, it is not a guaranteed form of birth control. The baby's frequent sucking while breastfeeding initiates the release of hormones that appear to suspend menstruation and ovulation. However, it is possible to ovulate and become fertile before menstruation returns.

There are several effective, safe and inexpensive forms of birth control that can be used, for example, natural family planning which involves the daily charting of fertility signs, such as basal body temperature, consistency of the cervical mucus, as well as the newest hand-held microscopes that show you visually, using your saliva, your personal ovulation cycle. These hand-held microscopes can be purchased at any drug store in North America. You can also use condoms or a diaphragm with spermicidal foam or jelly. Do not use oral contraceptives while breastfeeding.

Planning for a Homebirth

Excerpted from Informed Home Birth Magazine, *1995, written by Rahima Baldwin Dancy, founder of the Informed Homebirth and the Informed Birth & Parenting Association.*

Some medical people feel that women selfishly choose homebirth by putting their own experience above the safety of the baby. This is simply not true, everyone wants a healthy mother and a healthy baby. Couples who have their baby at home know that statistics bear out the safety of assisted homebirth for low-risk mothers; they also recognize that there are many advantages for the baby as well as the mother and the entire family.

Advantages for the baby include that she or he is more likely to be born vaginally, without the breathing difficulties often caused by cesarean birth or anesthesia. There is less likelihood of infection when the baby is with the mother than in the newborn nursery. The baby's experience at birth can be recognized and made as gentle as possible. Routine procedures such as deep suctioning, suctioning the stomach, scrubbing the baby, vitamin K shots, eye ointments and the like can be avoided.

Advantages for the mother include not being subjected to routine procedures such as electronic monitoring, IVs, shave, prep, enema or stirrups. She can eat and walk freely, her body working with nature. She will have continuity of care with the same attendants, increasing her safety. She is more likely to be treated and her progress evaluated as an individual, rather than being sacrificed to protocols or averages. She is much less likely to need pain killing drugs, forceps or a cesarean section when she has attendants who feel that birth is a normal physical function. She is comfortable in her own surroundings, relaxed and able to labor and deliver in the same place. She has less chance of infection and episiotomy. Postpartum depression is more uncommon since there are no unnecessary interventions or separation.

Advantages for the family include husbands in their own home rather than someone allowing them to be present. They can participate as fully as they want. Other children can be present as appropriate. A homebirth becomes an integral part of family life, helping to ease postpartum adjustment for all members of the family.

Shopping Tips

This is a good time to being assembling your layette. You can cut the cost of your layette in half by purchasing many of the items your baby will need second hand. Most infant clothing is only worn a few months and can easily go through a number of babies. Go to garage sales. Ask friends and family for items they no longer have use for. Look for second hand and consignment stores in your city for good quality clothing at excellent prices. To get the best value for your money buy most of your baby's clothing after your baby arrives. It is easy to buy too much in the wrong sizes.

If you find a mother to purchase clothing and baby accessories from stay in touch with her and call her two or three times a year to see if she has anything else she would like to sell. Talk to other mothers about what they found to be invaluable to have for the baby and what things they really didn't need. Purchase your crib and car seat new or nearly new. These two products are continually updated each year to provide our babies with the best in safety. Support the manufacturers in updating these products by buying your crib and car seat new, your newborn deserves the best in these two safety products.

Sample Layette Purchase
1 Dozen One Piece Undershirts
1 Dozen One Piece Jumpers
6 Large Flannel Receiving Blankets
4 Booties/Socks
1 Sweater/Hat
1 Snow Suit or Coat
2 Crib Sheets/2 Waterproof Pads/1 Bumper Pad
1 Quilt/Bassinet mattress and bedding
6 Washcloths
Baby Dove Soap
Johnson's Baby Body Wash
Baby Brush and Comb
Q-Tips for Umbilical Cord Care only. Never use Q-tips in your baby's ear as you can easily puncture the ear drum or push accumulated wax even further into the ear canal. Use a drop or two of mineral oil and a small piece of cotton to gently remove excess wax from the outside of the ear.
Rubbing Alcohol or Saline Solution for Umbilical Cord Care
Thermometer – Digital Ear Thermometers or underarm thermometers are best.
Nail File and Clippers
Sponge Bath Rest
A & D Creme for diaper rash and sore and cracked nipples
Diaper Pail
4 Dozen Prefolded Cloth Diapers

Size One Disposable Diapers for Travelling – Newborn size is often too small.

4 Pair Breathable Nylon (Not Plastic) Waterproof Pants with velcro attachments.

Hot/Cold Gel Packs for Breast Engorgement – Shoppers Drug Mart stores have the best hours of operation for new moms, many of their stores are open 24 hours offering great convenience for new mothers, and you will find an excellent selection of baby goods in every store.

Your layette for the first year may also include: Crib & Mattress, (not necessary if you use a family bed or bassinet), Change Table, Chest of Drawers, Infant Car Seat, Carriage or Stroller, High Chair, Safety Gate, Baby Swing, Rocking Chair, Sling, Breastfeeding Pillow, and assorted toys and books. Toy's R Us carries an excellent selection of everything that every baby needs. Baby products at this store are always well-displayed and easy to access.

You can reduce your costs by shopping smart, breastfeeding instead of bottle-feeding, and using cloth diapers instead of disposables. If you are unsure of whether you prefer cloth or disposable diapers, hire a diaper service for the first two months. As a new client you can usually ask for two weeks free. A diaper service with pick-up and drop-off once a week, is convenient, hassle-free, ecological and an excellent service for any mother. Services such as Stork Diaper Service charge about $15.00 per week. Today's pre-folded cloth diapers are quickly and easily changed with velcro strips instead of pins and breathable outer nylon covers instead of plastic pants. Cloth diapers are kinder on your baby's bottom and on the environment. Many mothers are now using both cloth and disposable diapers. A diaper service also saves you from that mad dash to the store for something you will need everyday for the first two years.

The Bay Department stores have an excellent selection of baby goods and they also stock the excellent Kooshies cloth diaper line. Cloth diapers reduce the number and types of rashes your baby may have from using disposable diapers and they can save you money from buying expensive prescription creams. Adding Borax to the wash cycle will help to keep the cloth diapers odor free and sanitized. When laundering your cloth diapers dissolve Borax into the water before adding diapers and then allow them to soak. This will change the acidic nature of the diaper to an alkaline nature. Borax can be found at Canada Safeway and London Drug stores. You may find it convenient to use both cloth and alternative disposable diapers. You can now purchase chemical-free disposable cotton diapers. In Canada, call Tushies at 1-888-720-2027.

Undershirts with attached bottoms are an excellent buy and most will last through three months of growing. You will find this to be the best uniform for your baby as they absorb leakage and keep your baby warm all over. Look for the Snugaby brand or Baby's Choice for excellent cotton, great durability and colors. These undershirts and flannel receiving blankets make the best baby uniform if you need to save money on clothing purchases having an abundance of both on hand makes it easy to clean up burps and spills.

What You Need To Know Before You Have Your Baby: The Best Care for A Premature Baby

Excerpted from Kangaroo Care: The Best You Can Do To Help Your Preterm Infant *by Susan M. Ludington-Hoe PhD with Susan K. Golant, 1993.*

Kangaroo Care, a program of skin-to-skin contact between parent and child, is part of the revolution in the care of premature infants. First researched in Latin America, Kangaroo Care was tested around the world during the 1980's and it is quickly becoming a popular treatment for premature infants. Neonatologists are seeing great improvements in newborns who participate in Kangaroo Care. Not only do the sleeping and breathing patterns of premature infants improve, the babies appear to relax and become content from the touch of their parents' skin. Parents also benefit psychologically because they are allowed to play an active rather than a passive role in the recovery of their infant.

Scores of international scientific studies have shown that Kangaroo Care offers the preterm infant many physical and emotional benefits. These benefits include:

A more stable heart rate.

More regular breathing.

Improved dispersion of oxygen throughout the body.

Prevention of cold stress.

Longer periods of sleep during which the brain matures.

More rapid weight gain.

Reduction of purposeless activity which simply burns calories at the expense of the infant's growth and health.

Decreased crying.

Longer periods of alertness.

Opportunities to breastfeed.

Greater opportunities for both parents and infant to attach.

Increased likelihood of being discharged from the hospital sooner.

The benefits to parents have also been well documented. Those who have practiced Kangaroo Care feel more positive about the birth experience despite its inherent difficulty. They are eager and ready to bring their babies home and feel confident in handling them because they have already enjoyed opportunities to create a loving relationship. This is true of fathers as well as mothers. In short, Kangaroo Care helps premature babies to recover as it enables their parents to lovingly, actively, and positively participate in their care.

Easy Steps for Kangaroo Care

Get yourself ready by having a meal and emptying your bladder as you'll be sitting for a one or two hour period. If you have a cold or the flu postpone the session until you're absolutely well, unless you are in a private room or at home. Your baby will be protected but the others may not. Make sure you are well away from any drafts or hot sunny windows. A large chair with arm rests and a foot rest will give you the best support. Use a telephone book, boxes, stool or whatever else is at hand. If the chair is not equipped with a foot rest elevate your legs to half the height of the chair to ensure good circulation in your legs.

Your infant must not be totally naked under any circumstances. First, he should be wearing a diaper to protect both of you from becoming wet. Moisture will have a cooling effect on your skin and his skin. A standard preemie diaper is often too large on a very small baby. If you do use one make sure it is folded down so skin contact can occur from his belly button up. Try a surgical mask instead of the diaper for a really small baby.

Purchase a soft, lined woolen hat rather than using the standard issue stockinette cap given by the hospital. The greatest heat loss in your baby is lost through the head. A new flannel receiving blanket works best to cover your baby. Start with the blanket folded in fourths. Should your baby become too warm, first take off the headcap and booties, and then you can unfold the blanket once and then twice.

Tiny or sick babies may be unable to keep their chests expanded during upright Kangaroo Care. If your preemie is under 32 weeks and weighs less than 1,500 grams or if she is very sick, you will need to hold her in a more reclined position. Angle her so that she's resting on one breast or the other. Also use a blanket that has been previously warmed. If your baby is still on a ventilator, recruit two staff members to assist you in getting your baby into position. Your chair must be close enough to the equipment so that the wires and tubes are not pulled or stretched. Have everything set up with you in the chair before you arrange the transfer. A semi-reclined position is best for both of you, allowing your baby's head to be turned in one direction or the other so that the ventilator tubes and gadgetry rest on your shoulder.

Place your baby, skin-to-skin, on your chest placing your baby in the fetal position, arms and legs bent and tucked beneath the torso to help conserve your baby's heat. Your breast will heat up or cool down your baby automatically as needed. Close access to your breast will give your baby the most practice with breastfeeding. Your baby will eventually suck and rest and suck and rest as needed. Ask for special assistance from your health team as premature infants have common problems with breastfeeding that can be easily remedied with help.

Stay in place for as long as you feel comfortable. Even thirty minutes of Kangaroo Care can have a tremendous positive impact on both you and your baby. Expect your baby to fall into a long deep sleep. You may want to use this time to nap as well. Most sessions last an hour or two. Some mothers are choosing to wear their babies day and night for the first month or so with excellent results for both parents and baby.

Enlist the support of your partner. Men receive the same benefits as we do and are often surprised at their own nurturing abilities and they begin to feel deeply attached to their tiny babies. The best time to begin Kangaroo Care is immediately after birth. Talk to your health team about this great new advance in premature care and let them know of your intention to Kangaroo Care your baby. You may want to work on changing the environment of your hospital's Intensive Care Nursery to further help your baby to sleep and grow:

1. Ask to have the lights dimmed.
2. Have the radio turned off and have your baby placed furthest away from traffic.
3. Ask for a smaller private or semi-private room for your baby.
4. Have the nurse put up a "Please do not disturb me. This is my nap time" at designated times of the day and night that you choose.
5. Make a sleep shade (like a sun shade) to help facilitate your baby's day-night cycling. Allow it to cover the top and two sides of the incubator but leave open the ends from which the wires emerge.
6. Create a nest for your baby within the incubator or crib. You can use bolsters of fabric that are at least as high as his body. There are various ways of creating these bolsters. You can use rolled blankets, foam forms, rubber doughnuts, a hammock, Neocrate by Snugli or even a bean bag that you've made the size of your baby and covered with a soft natural fabric.
7. Ask the hospital to have a "nursery shutdown" when all babies are given a long opportunity to sleep undisturbed.

Nursery shutdown, reduced lighting, and sleep shades are examples of conditions you can implement or advocate to protect your infant from the stressful NICU environment. Distancing your baby from sudden loud noises and nesting her will reduce her agitation. Day-night cycling, prone position, and nesting all foster better sleep as does Kangaroo Care. Kangaroo Care also has the potent role of replacing noxious experiences with pleasant loving ones.

8

Eighth Month

As your baby becomes heavier, make sure you take every opportunity to sit rather than stand. Do not lift heavy items. Take the elevator instead of the stairs and continue to remind those around you that you are pregnant and these activities are not advised.

Keep a supply of ice cubes and crushed ice to suck on. You can also freeze lemonade in your ice cube trays.

Anyone who offers to help now in the first few days after your baby's arrival – accept! Even having a load of laundry done or the house tidied up a bit is a wonderful break. Also having someone to chat with will help you to recuperate emotionally as well. Ask what they do best and book them in advance. Remember you should be handling your baby, as parenting is practice. Have your helpers take care of the one hundred and one other tasks that need to be done.

Gardening is a great stress reliever and squatting while weeding strengthens your thighs and pelvic floor, to assist you with the pushing phase of your delivery.

Try to relax! Take time out each and every day to do something for yourself. Your body needs time to rest and sometimes a nap is not always possible (especially if you have older children or if you are working throughout your pregnancy). Time for yourself is very important for your health and your state of mind.

Breastfeeding Clinics

Plan to attend a breastfeeding class or a La Leche support group now in your neighborhood. It is important that you find out how to breastfeed your baby before birth. There is a lot of information that can make your breastfeeding experience a success for you both right from the start. Meet the instructor so you will always have someone to call upon should the need arise. The Childbirth Resource Directory has listings for both Canada and the United

States headquarters. These toll-free numbers will direct you to the nearest neighborhood meeting. Most of the moms who volunteer with this organization overcame some challenges themselves during breastfeeding and usually have great empathy for any concerns or questions you may have.

Preventing Postnatal Depression

Purchase extra prenatal vitamins from your health food store. You will need to continue your vitamins for at least ninety days after your baby is born.

Stock up your cupboards and freezer with easy to prepare meals and high-energy snack foods. Prepare to have enough food put away for your first two weeks of rest. Arrange for a caretaker for yourself for the two weeks. You will require someone to prepare food, take trips to the drug store and grocery store, and to watch the baby while you take walks outside, bath or sleep.

Drugs used to induce or speed up your labor can cause prolonged postnatal depression. Avoid these drugs during childbirth for this reason alone.

The more assistance you have the first two weeks, the less severe any depression will be. You may be better off having a female than a male for this, as a woman is more likely to anticipate your needs. Make sure you arrange for a back-up caregiver as well. Have your partner take time off after the first month or two when your baby will be more awake and alert.

Plan to have telephone contact with someone who knows you throughout your first month home. Depression can silently sneak up on you and those who know you well will become aware of it often before you realize that you are depressed.

It is important to grieve for what you have lost; independence, money, time for your own interests, self-care, freedom to come and go as you please or whatever you feel is missing from your life now. You may also be grieving the end of your pregnancy. Then be mindful of what you have gained in exchange.

Some days will be easier than others.

Make sure you are continuing to take your prenatal vitamins. B vitamins are extremely helpful in combating depression.

St. John's Wort, an extract from a flower, is the newest natural product to assist in healing postnatal depression. It can be purchased at any health food store in capsules, drops or oil. Taking 300 milligrams three times a day has given many women quick relief from depression. It is a natural and non-toxic product and can be taken while you continue breastfeeding.

Leritone "Vitality" can also help to naturally heal depression and end sluggish thinking. This product has been on the market for over twenty years and it can be found at most health food stores. Take 2 to 4 capsules once a day, preferably in the morning before food. You may notice a marked difference in the first week of taking it.

Liquid, colloidal minerals supplemented daily will give your body extra support if your depression has been triggered by nutritional exhaustion.

Talk to other women who have just had babies. You will be surprised to find out that they are having many of the same feelings that you are.

If you had a bad experience during your birth find a way to heal this. One of the best ways is to vent your feelings to your health team. Let them know what you feel they could have done differently. You may not be able to change your experience, but you may change the experience of those who come after you. In Canada or the United States, contact the College of Physicians and Surgeons listed in the white pages of your telephone directory to voice your complaint and request a disciplinary hearing. You do not need a lawyer to bring a complaint to the College. Writing a letter is often sufficient to bring much needed changes into the system.

Talk about your feelings with those around you. Be ready to let others step in to help so that you can have time to yourself to rebalance. Make sure that you are getting out of the house on a regular basis to reconnect with your friends and family. Take up all offers for baby-sitting even if its just for an hour or two. This is extremely important if your baby has a colic condition and you find your sleep interrupted night after night all through the night.

This Isn't What I Expected: Recognizing and Recovering from Depression and Anxiety After Childbirth by Karen R. Mleiman, MSc, and Valerie D. Raskin, MD, is a book for the 1 out of 4 mothers who find life after a baby unexpectedly difficult for a variety of reasons. This book provides excellent information on how to recognize the signs, where to find help and everyday coping techniques. Several exercises are designed to help you explore your feelings about parenthood, how you were parented, and how your expectations have clashed with reality. The real-life stories help us to see ourselves through others and know that we are not alone.

If you feel that you can't cope, or if you have feelings of violence towards yourself or your baby, seek professional help immediately. Don't wait to feel better: if you have a clinical depression it will most likely get worse with time so deal with this situation right away. Your closest childbirth association, doctor or midwife will be able to direct you to an agency that has experience with postnatal depression.

Preparing for a Faster and Easier Labor

You may be able to avoid the pain of back labor during delivery by assisting your baby to turn to the proper placement, head down and facing back, by going on your hand and knees in the evening and gently rocking your hips back and forth. Place your knees apart to open up the pelvic area. You can also lean against an ottoman or the sofa if this is more comfortable. This position will help by giving your baby more room to turn around and this position is soothing for yourself as well. A ten-minute session of this every other night is plenty.

Visualize your baby actually turning in your womb, head down with the face back. Every time you go in for your prenatal appointments look at your doctor's charts and models of babies to clearly see the position your baby will need to be into for an easy birth. If your heath team says your baby has dropped and you still have a few weeks to go until your due date – celebrate! The longer your baby is "engaged" the more pliable your body becomes. A little pressure for a longer time will make dilating during active labor quicker and easier. Some babies to not "drop" until the last few moments of delivery, so don't be concerned if you don't feel this happening.

Child Care

Put an ad into your local paper for a high school or college student. Screen applicants carefully over the telephone. Look for a high school student in your neighborhood, or a college student with a car. Ask for expected hourly salary, experience with newborns, references and get a feel for who they are over the telephone. It will give you peace of mind knowing you have an alternate caregiver even if you don't use her right away. Interview in person the best three candidates and call all references.

Begin to investigate your child care options. A live-out nanny can easily cost $7.00 per hour with paid statutory holidays. If you have an established career; you may decide that a nanny is the best value for your money. Picking up and dropping off your baby to a sitter or daycare can easily take two productive hours out of your day. Having dinner prepared by someone else can add an hour to your day.

An established day-care center may charge from $400 to $500 per month. All day-care centers have a limit of infants that they can accept, so booking ahead will help with this. Some day-care centers offer subsidies from the government which can reduce the amount you pay. Ask in advance about subsidies and fill out the necessary paperwork so that you have it on hand. Home day-care centers often charge from $20.00 to $30.00 per day. Overtime hours are often charged at double, so make sure you are clear about this at the start. Taking the time now to investigate what is offered in your city will help you to make calm, clear decisions after your baby arrives.

Take a look at the amount you actually bring in from working after taxes, day-care, transportation, lunches, extra clothing expenses and all costs associated with working. Are you actually getting ahead? Studies are now showing that the first three years of your baby's life is the most critical period of time when you can make the greatest impact in your baby's life. This is the time when your baby will develop the framework and foundation of who he or she will become. Giving up some material benefits now in exchange for this extremely important time in your baby's life may be the most rewarding option you can choose.

Siblings

Spend time with older children prior to your baby's arrival discussing what it will be like to have a new baby in the house. Many children think they will have a ready-to-play friend arriving. The older children need to understand that babies eat, sleep, cry and take up a lot of Mom and Dad's time and energy in the first few months. Their expectations will be more realistic if they are prepared in advance for these events.

If you are planning a home birth or family-centered birth, explain that labor does hurt, and give them an idea of what the new baby will look like and act like at birth. Most children handle a home birth with tact and diplomacy and can provide great comfort to their mother during labor and birth. Allowing the children to come in and out of the room as they please and having a responsible adult on hand to care for them during the birth can help them to participate in this exciting day. Mothers who birth at home are reporting that there is less friction and sibling rivalry in the family due in great part to the children's involvement in the birth.

Planning a Waterbirth

Excerpted from The Waterbirth Handbook, *Dr. Roger Lichy and Eileen Herzberg, 1993.*

In the past decade or so, women from all walks of life have labored and given birth in such unusual water containers as a cattle trough in Texas, a skip in England and glass tanks in Russia. Women have given birth in hot springs and in the sea, in swimming pools, paddling pools, jacuzzis, in ordinary baths and purpose-built tubs all over the world. Waterbirths have captured women's imagination as a natural, safe and effective method of pain relief, as part of the trend towards natural childbirth. It's an idea whose time has come. Midwives have known about the soothing effects of warm water for generations. The first medically-recorded waterbirth took place in France in 1803. The birth attendants were at their wits' end to know what to do to help a woman deliver after she had been in hard labor for forty-eight hours. One of the midwives suggested a warm bath, hoping that it might ease her pain. Almost as soon as the exhausted woman got into the bath the baby was born.

Waterbirth seminars are being organized for midwives and doctors and more hospitals are providing facilities for waterbirths. Research has begun to provide evidence and statistics. Women's enthusiasm for waterbirths is helping to make them more widely available and there's growing official recognition that women should be offered the choice of using water in labor and childbirth. For example, in England, the House of Commons Health Committee on Maternity Services has recommended that hospitals provide birthing pool facilities. Since 1993, more than 70 hospitals in Great Britain provide pool facilities to birthing mothers. It's an option that is increasingly available to women in hospitals, homes and birthing centers around the world.

The relaxing effects of water reduce pain during labor and delivery by causing the mother to have a lower heart rate and blood pressure, lower respiratory rate, lower blood lactic acid levels, a decrease in oxygen consumption, lower muscle tone, lower blood cortisone levels, increase in perfusion of internal organs, increase in skin temperature and causes an increase in the electrical resistance of skin.

Warm water also helps the uterine muscle to work more efficiently, it relieves uncomfortable positions, boosts pain relieving endorphins, lowers stress hormones and relaxes pelvic floor muscles helping to stretch the birth canal without tearing and for dialation to occur at a faster rate. Any gentle childbirth will enable you and your baby to feel relaxed and peaceful as you get to know each other, but water does seem to add an extra dimension, a stronger sense of serenity. This may be the effect of the potent emotional, spiritual and symbolic quality of water because in both a literal and symbolic sense, water is the mother of us all. Literally, life on earth first evolved from the sea and, symbolically, water is widely recognized as epitomizing birth and rebirth. Baptism in water represents rebirth, traditional Chinese medicine calls water the mother of life and Freudian psychotherapists interpret water as both birth and the mother.

Dr. Lichy goes on to cover every aspect of water birthing including its fascinating history, safety, choice of tubs and how to book a water birth as well as useful advice on how to make the most of water throughout labor and during delivery. This book is filled with photographs of calm, alert babies and their mothers. *The Waterbirth Handbook* is a fascinating documentary on the benefits of water birth.

Natural Remedies for Yeast Infections

Clear your body of excess yeast now if you are having persistent yeast infections. During the course of any treatment for vaginal yeast it is important to cut out sugar and decrease dairy and bread consumption. Purchase any generic bottle of acidophilus capsules (our friendly bacteria), from the cooler in your health food store. Take 2 tablets vaginally for 3 nights before you sleep and take 2 capsules orally a day with your evening meal. If you are prone to yeast infections continue to take the acidophilus capsules orally until the end of your pregnancy and for the first few months of breastfeeding. Always store acidophilus in your refrigerator.

Excess yeast in your system can be transferred to your baby through the birth canal. Yeast can cause thrush in a newborn and will cause problems with breastfeeding. Thrush shows up as white patches inside your baby's mouth and your nipples become extremely sensitive and sore, making breastfeeding difficult and painful. Should thrush become a problem during breastfeeding you and your baby will both have to be treated to eliminate it and the drugs available for this treatment are extremely expensive. As always with any challenge you may experience during breast-feeding, call a La Leche Leader or a Lactation Consultant at your nearest hospital. Always consult other women who have breastfed for breastfeeding challenges. You need someone who has personal experience. The La Leche leaders are always only a phone call away.

If your yeast infection persists see your doctor for alternate treatment. Some vaginal infections may mimic yeast symptoms but may actually be trichomonas, bacterial vaginosis, gonorrhea, chlamydia or even herpes. A quick test by your doctor can easily show you the cause of the infection.

Excerpted from: Take Charge of Your Body, *Dr. Carolyn DeMarco, Fifth Edition, 1994.*

In 1973, on my first day of work as a medical doctor, a woman walked into my office having suffered from vaginal itching for 20 years. She turned out to have a chronic yeast infection, which eventually she was able to overcome. At various times throughout their lives, many women experience one or more vaginal infections. These highly annoying and even painful infections usually clear up rapidly with treatment. However, an estimated 20% of women go on to develop persistent and recurrent yeast infections.

Of course, the female body has its own defences against invading yeast cells. The vagina itself is a balanced ecosystem. It is an efficient, self-maintaining and dynamic environment with natural defence mechanisms that keep it healthy, moist and clean. The two most important defence mechanisms are the acid base balance and the cervical secretions. This acid condition of the vagina discourages infections by bacteria and other organisms. Friendly bacteria called lactobacillus acidophilus also help to keep the vagina acidic and resistant to infections.

Certain predisposing factors for yeast infections include use of a birth control pill, pregnancy, use of antibiotics, steroid or anti-cancer drugs, diabetes, the overall state of your health and menopause. Predisposing factors that can also cause recurring yeast infections include warm moist conditions, tight or synthetic clothing, deodorants and sprays, perfumed tampons, perfumed toilet paper, bubble baths with chemicals or perfumes, douching, (pregnant women should never douche), improper toilet habits, vaginal abrasions and sex. Yeast probably can be sexually transmitted, but this has not yet been proven.

However, in a large percentage of cases, yeast can also be cultured from the penises of men whose partners have recurrent yeast infections. In these cases, the men may need to take oral anti-yeast medications while their partners are being treated. Even for simple yeast infections, condoms should be used until the woman has completed her treatment.

The main symptoms of yeast infections are usually vaginal discharge and itching of the genital area. The discharge is usually white and varies from being a little to a lot; from being thin and mucousy to thick, curdy and cottage cheese-like with anything in between being possible. The amount of itching also varies but can be severe enough to interfere with sleep and normal activities. Some women notice a characteristic odor suggestive of bread dough or the fermenting yeast smell of beer. Other frequent symptoms are swelling, redness and irritation of the outer and inner lips, the labia, painful sex or painful urination due to local irritation of the urethra.

A woman with a full-blown yeast infection is acutely uncomfortable and requires immediate treatment if possible. If you suspect that you have a yeast infection see your doctor as soon as possible in order to get cultures of the vaginal secretions taken. Other vaginal infections can co-exist or produce a similar picture of signs and symptoms.

After you have had yeast infection confirmed by culture, or while waiting to see your doctor, you can begin treatment right away with some simple over the counter remedies. An old remedy that is effective against both yeast and trichomonas is the use of a clove of garlic. The garlic is peeled but not nicked, and wrapped in gauze making a kind of tampon with a gauze tail. The garlic is inserted vaginally and left in place for twelve hours. The treatment usually goes on for three days. For relief of itching try witch hazel compresses, warm water baths with Epsom salts or baking soda, or a poultice of cottage cheese on a sanitary napkin. Other natural anti-yeast preparations include a new and highly effective preparation of grapefruit seed extract in doses of five to fifteen drops three or four times a day taken orally in juice for five to nine months. This extract is sold as "Nutri-Biotic," a liquid concentrate that can be purchased at drug and health food stores.

Persistent and recurrent yeast infections may be part of a larger picture involving widespread overgrowth of yeast organisms in the whole body. This may cause symptoms affecting every system of the body which may include fatigue, depression, digestive difficulties, menstrual problems, sexual difficulties and infertility, arthritis, chronic skin problems, repeated urinary and vaginal infections, asthma, allergic reactions and chemical sensitivities. Candida overgrowth may also be suspected when a person feels very ill and no cause can be found for his or her problems. Women are particularly susceptible to candida overgrowth, especially if they have been exposed to tetracycline for treatment of acne or long-term use of the birth control pill. In children, a chronic yeast infection can show up as hyperactivity, learning disabilities, or even in a few cases autism. In adolescents, candida can cause depression and severe mood swings. A typical story is a top student who suddenly becomes unable to think clearly or learn, and who becomes suicidally depressed. In one teenage girl these symptoms appeared after just a two-month course of tetracycline for acne. Candida has also been implicated in some cases of teenage anorexia.

If you suspect this generalized type of candida problem, the first step should be to visit your doctor for a complete history and physical examination including appropriate blood tests to rule out other possible causes of your symptoms as low thyroid function, other glandular abnormalities, anemia, low blood sugar, viral infections or parasitic infections. It is important to remember that each of these conditions can mimic chronic yeast infections or co-exist with them.

The next step involves educating yourself about candida in its many and varied manifestations. Six books are recommended:

The Yeast Syndrome by Dr. J.P. Trowbridge and M. Walker, 1986
Back to Health by Dr. D.W. Remington and B.W. Higa, 1987
The Missing Diagnosis by Dr. C.O. Truss 1985
The Yeast Connection by Dr. William Crook, 1989
Candida by Dr. Luc DeShepper, 1986
Who Killed Candida? by Vicki Glasburn, 1991

If the problem is detected in its early stages, treatment is much more successful. Treatment involves dietary and lifestyle changes as well as the use of either prescription or non-prescription anti-yeast medications on a long-term basis.

For more information you can contact:

Health Foundation, PO Box 3494, Jackson, TN 38303 (901) 427-8100

Yeast Consulting Services, PO Box 11157, Torrance, CA 905010, (310) 375-1073

Candida Research Information Service, 41 Green Valley Court, Kleinburg, Ontario, L0J 1C0, (416) 832-0789

The vagina has a wonderful built-in defence system. But in today's fast-paced lifestyle, with its over-reliance on drugs, poor diet and environmental stresses, natural defence systems may be overwhelmed. A simple yeast infection now and then is easy to treat but a chronic yeast infection requires a more thoughtful and thorough approach.

What You Need to Know before You Have Your Baby: New Effective Pain Relief for Labor & Delivery

Excerpted from Mothering Magazine, *Spring 1997, The Epidural Express: Real Reasons Not to Jump on Board, written by Nancy Griffin, MA, AAHCC. Nancy Griffin is a Bradley Method natural childbirth educator, a pregnancy-recovery exercise specialist, breastfeeding educator and the owner of Mommy Care Mothering Center in West L.A. USA 90025 (310) 394-6711. Her web site is http://www.yoyoweb.co/wospace.*

One of the most emotionally charged issues in childbirth is how to deal safely and effectively with pain during birth. Epidurals have become so commonplace that most hospitals automatically include them in their standard billing protocol for all vaginal deliveries. The epidural at first appeared to be a magic bullet for pain in childbirth. Many women are still told that the medication used in an epidural is completely safe and that it does not reach the baby. The passage of time, combined with new research has begun to reveal a different picture.

There are actually several kinds of epidurals. The type that most people refer to is, in fact, a lumbar epidural – the administration of a regional anesthetic agent, or a combination of an anesthetic agent with a narcotic and/or antihypertensive, which is injected into the lumbar region of the laboring woman's back by a qualified anesthetic care provider. It is performed by inserting a long needle into the epidural space of the spine, through which a soft catheter is threaded. The needle is then removed and the catheter taped in place. Doses of anesthetic can then be periodically or continuously administered through this catheter.

The mother must lie curled on her side without moving during this procedure, which takes from 20 to 30 minutes to complete and take effect. Once it is in effect, she will be numb from her ribs to her toes, and sensations of pain usually will be eliminated. Epidurals can be strong enough to provide complete loss of sensation and all pain during a cesarean, or minimal enough that the mother can still feel when to push in a vaginal birth. A "walking" epidural is a lumbar epidural in which the dosage of narcotics is higher and the regional anesthetic dosage is lower, creating pain relief without total numbness in the lower body.

The Physician's Desk Reference, a well-respected guide to all drugs, their usage, cautions, and side-effects, states the following about the canine derivatives used in epidurals: "Local anesthetics rapidly cross the placenta and when used for epidural blocks, anesthesia can cause varying degrees of maternal, fetal, and neonatal toxicity. Adverse reactions in the mother and baby involve alteration of the central nervous system, peripheral vascular tone and cardiac function. The following possible maternal side effects include hypotension, urinary retention, fecal and urinary incontinence, paralysis of lower extremities, headache, backache, septic meningitis, slowing of labor, increased need for forceps or vacuum delivery, cranial nerve palsies, allergic reactions, respiratory depression, nausea, vomiting and seizures."

Research done in the last five years on the effects of epidural anesthesia on newborns has shown that epidurals result in lowered neurobehavioral scores in the newborn; a decrease in muscle tone and strength, affecting the baby's sucking ability, which can lead to breastfeeding difficulties; respiratory depression in the baby; greater likelihood of fetal malpositioning; and an increase in fetal heart rate variability, thereby increasing the need for forceps, vacuum, and cesarean deliveries and episiotomies. A review of the literature reports that on average over 70% of women receiving an epidural during childbirth experience some side effects.

Very rare but possible risks of epidurals include trauma to nerve fibers if the epidural needle enters a nerve and the injection goes directly into that nerve; a drug overdose resulting in profound hypertension with respiratory and cardiac arrest and possible death; and central nervous system toxicity resulting from an injection directly into the epidural vein. Other medical interventions, such as IVs, continuous electronic fetal monitoring, the use of additional drugs, bladder catheterization, continuous administration of oxygen, and forceps, vacuum extraction, and episiotomies often become necessary as adjunct medical care to an epidural. Epidurals can prolong a labor leading to the possible need to augment labor with more drugs.

The Physician's Desk Reference repeatedly states that "no adequate and well-controlled studies exist for use of these drugs in pregnant women" and that "it is not known whether these drugs can cause fetal harm when administered to a pregnant woman." Many unnecessary epidurals are the result of a well-meaning health care provider telling the birthing mother that, "It's time for an epidural now." Women in labor are vulnerable, and often easily influenced by the attitudes of those around them. Dr. Jeffrey Illeck, an obstetrician at Cedars-Sinai Medical Center in Los Angeles feels that routine epidurals have "become a way of making the nurse's job in large hospitals easier therefore increasing the number of epidurals that occur. Nurses are extremely busy and often have lost their skills to coach a woman in labor." He also states that, "A lot of the problem is the patient's fear and helping them through these fears."

Anything causing fear in the birthing mother will increase her pain. Despite the fact that we have technology at our disposal, our biology provides us with powerful instincts during birth. The first is the need to feel safe and protected. All mammals will instinctively seek out a dark, secluded, quiet, and most of all, safe place in which to give birth. While birthing, mammals give the appearance of sleep and closed eyes to fool would-be predators, and they breathe normally. Some, those who don't perspire, will pant in order to cool down, but humans will most easily achieve a relaxed state through closed eyes and abdominal breathing. This relaxation slows down the birthing mother's brain waves into what is called an alpha state, a state in which it is virtually impossible to release adrenaline, the "fright-flight" hormone. Physical comfort becomes critical, along with the need to have a nest ready for the baby.

Hospital environments often unintentionally disrupt the birthing atmosphere by introducing bright lights, lots of people, noise, and fear-inducing exams and machines. Put it all together and you have fear, and therefore stress, and stress causes pain. The uterine muscles are beautifully designed to deal quite effectively with danger, fear, and stress in labor. The uterus is the only muscle in the body that contains within itself two, opposing muscle groups – one to induce and continue labor and another to stop labor if the birthing mother is in danger or afraid.

Emotional or physical stress will automatically signal danger to a birthing mammal. Her labor will slow down or stop completely so that she can run to safety. In modern times, this goes haywire. We can't run from our fears. Instead, we may release adrenaline, which causes the short, circular muscle fibers in the lower third of the uterus to contract. These muscles are responsible for stopping labor by closing and tightening the cervix. The result is that we literally stew in our own adrenaline. At the same time that the long, straight muscle fibers of the uterus are contracting to efface and dilate the cervix, the short, circular muscle fibers of the lower uterus are also contracting to keep the cervix closed and fight the labor. The result? The very real pain of two powerful muscles pulling in opposite directions each time the birthing mother has a contraction. The constant presence of a loving, supportive, and trained labor coach, effective education about the birthing process, and a health team and environment the birthing mother can trust can make all the difference in the world.

Unnecessary or preventable pain can also be caused during labor by simple things such as prohibiting the laboring mother from walking, changing position, or moving around freely according to her instincts. Freedom of movement literally supports rotation and alignment, the process by which the baby turns and moves down through the pelvic inlet and outlet. Time-honored birthing traditions have always included walking, changing positions, rocking, and even floating in water. Anything that assists the rotation and alignment of the baby during labor will automatically improve the efficiency of contractions, thereby shortening labor and decreasing pain.

Avoiding unnecessary medical interventions during labor will decrease pain because these interventions actually cause pain themselves, leading to routine epidurals. The use of routine interventions interferes with the natural process of birth, which is inherently safe and effective. How is it possible to know whether medical interventions are unnecessary? The answer is surprisingly simple. If both mother and baby are doing fine during labor, they're unnecessary.

Proper and adequate nutrition during pregnancy and eating and drinking to appetite and thirst during labor can also dramatically decrease pain. Inadequate consumption of complex carbohydrates and water during labor can result in dehydration and low blood sugar, both of which cause more painful and less effective contractions.

A safe and effective exercise program during pregnancy should include aerobic conditioning to provide the mother with needed endurance during labor, as well as pregnancy-specific exercises, which include Kegels, pelvic rocking, and squatting to prepare her body physically for labor. When the mother's body is strong and prepared, pain is decreased. She will have the strength and endurance for pushing in second stage labor, perhaps decreasing the length of the pushing stage and thereby decreasing pain.

Pain During Transition – Choose a position that feels right, relax completely and surrender to and trust the birth process. Use counter-pressure if needed and assure the laboring mother that she is almost through.

Back Labor – Use a hands-and-knees position with your labor coach providing counter-pressure on the painful spot. Walking and changing positions can help to rotate the baby out of the posterior position relieving back labor completely.

Crowning – Nature makes the most difficult moments the shortest. Crowning rarely lasts longer than one to three pushes in an unmedicated birth. By choosing her own birthing position and avoiding the traditional hospital pushing positions, the mother can make crowning far less painful. Squatting widens the pelvic outlet by up to 28% in a pregnant woman and utilizes gravity to assist the birth. Your health care professional can also provide perineal massage or support during the delivery.

Once women are educated about epidurals it becomes clear that avoiding one during childbirth may be well worth it to both mother and baby. By taking responsibility for her health and the health of her baby long before labor begins there are a great many things a mother can do to tremendously improve her chances of successfully avoiding an epidural.

9

Homestretch

Review your birth plan. Have it kept in your medical file and discuss it thoroughly with your health care specialists. If you do not reach agreement on your plan, or if you feel uncertain that it will be complied with, it's not too late to change to another caregiver. Make sure you feel confident about your caregiver, follow your instincts completely in this matter, do not let any health professional intimidate you.

If you have time at home prior to delivering, get a few things organized for your baby. It goes without saying that your baby's room needs to be prepared and purchases made in that department by now like the crib, clothing items, car seat, receiving blankets and quilts. However, some people forget the obvious, simple things, like diapers, wipes, and cremes.

Cook ahead! If you have a freezer it is a good idea to get some meals or baking done up ahead of time. Think of yourself being snowed in for a month and plan accordingly. There will be some days during recovery when getting supper to the table will be nearly impossible.

If you are making an announcement in the newspaper, write it up in draft form using the ones in the paper as examples. Then you can just fill in the blanks! Call your newspaper to get rates, deadlines, etc.

If you plan to send announcement cards, buy them ahead and address the envelopes. You can fill in the cards once you have the details. Thank you cards can also be purchased ahead of time so that you can send them to people as the gifts come in. It is rather daunting to have to write 20 or 30 cards all at once. You may find that after your baby arrives you will be too distracted and tired to start from scratch on projects like these.

Go to your health food store and purchase more red raspberry leaf tea. Red raspberry leaf tea will help to condition your uterus for the work it will need to do in the next few weeks. You can use any left-over tea after your baby is born to help shrink your uterus back to its original size.

You'll find a nightly warm bath in clear water a lifesaver for this time of your pregnancy. A bath relaxes tense and strained muscles, soothes away aches and pains and has a very calming effect on both you and your baby. You will also enjoy the feelings of weightlessness.

Short walks by yourself can provide you with the comfort of fresh air, exercise and a great chance to "work out" negative thoughts and become more comfortable with your pregnant body and the baby soon to come.

Find a beauty salon or school offering a package deal for facial, manicure and pedicure. Reward yourself – you deserve it.

Packing Your Bag

Labor is hard work. Keep your body well nourished on this day. Clothes you will be needing include heavy socks or slippers for walking, a housecoat, a sweat suit with extra pants to wear home, and perhaps an oversized T-shirt for laboring in. Buy a T-shirt with a funny saying on it to remind you to keep your sense of humor and to keep as a great momento. This is infinitely better than any hospital gown ever designed.

Bring high-energy foods such as a nut mix, chocolate, yogurt, soup and sandwiches and plenty to drink like herbal teas, juice, and non-caffeinated pop. A recipe for Labor-Aid is included in the next section, mix up a batch for you and your partner. A disposable camera with flash, your birth plan, one sleeper for baby with hat, large baby blanket and an infant carseat is needed.

A surprise bag with a tape deck or Walkman with your favorite music, a favorite photograph, and a pillow and blanket can make your room more comfortable and will also help you with the various stages of your labor. Bring a slow-cooking crock pot, an unopened bottle of vegetable oil, like olive oil and some cloth compresses to apply the oil or heated water.

Pack some pain control techniques you have written on separate pieces of paper and placed into an envelope. Have your partner put some jokes or funny sayings in there. Throughout your labor take one out and do what you've written every so often, for example: Use Picture / Play Music / Shower / Walk / Massage / Jokes / Loose Lips = Loose Cervix (Dilation occurs faster when mouth is relaxed) = Time for a Kiss / Anything else you can think of.

Shopping Tips

If your baby will have older siblings you may want to prepare them by having them buy a small gift for the baby – a blanket or rattle for example. In turn, your baby can buy a small item for them such as a book, healthy goodies or crayons. Your new baby will probably be receiving a lot of attention and gifts so it helps to even things out and help the siblings feel included. It also helps to have the older brother or sister open the baby gifts as they come in.

Purchase a hot/cold gel pack and well as aspirin or Tylenol for fever when your breastmilk comes in. A Playtex nursing set is great to have on hand as the plastic bags come in handy when you begin to store and freeze your breastmilk. Going to the drug store at 3:00 in the morning for this essential equipment is disheartening with a full fever. Pick up some heavy flow sanitary napkins as well as you may go through at least two or three packages after your baby is born.

BIRTH

Once upon a time, twins were conceived in the womb. Seconds, minutes, hours passed as the two dormant lives developed. The spark of life flowed until it fanned fire with the formation of their embryonic brains. With their simple brains came feeling, and with feeling, perception, a perception of surroundings, of each other, of self.

When they perceived the life of each other and their own life, they knew that life was good, and they laughed and rejoiced; the one saying, "Lucky are we to have been conceived, and to have this world," and the other chiming, "Blessed be the Mother who gave us this life and each other."

Each budded and grew arms and fingers, legs and toes. They stretched their hands and churned and turned in their new-found world. They explored their worlds, and in it found the life cord which gave them life from the precious Mother's blood. So they sang, "How great is the love of the Mother that she shares all she has with us!" And they were pleased and satisfied with their lot.

Weeks passed into months, and with the advent of each new month, they noticed a change in each other and each began to see change in himself. "We are changing," said the one. "What can it mean?"

"It means," replied the other, "that we are drawing near to birth."

An unsettling chill crept over the two, and they both feared, for they knew that birth meant leaving all their world behind.

Said the one, "Were it up to me, I would live here forever."

"We must be born," said the other.

"It has happened to all others who were here." For indeed there was evidence of life there before, as the Mother had borne others.

"But mightn't there be life after birth?"

"How can there be life after birth?" cried the one. "Do we not shed our life cord and also the blood tissue? And have you ever talked to one that has been born? Has anyone ever re-entered the womb after birth? No!" He fell into despair, and in his despair he moaned, "If the purpose of conception and all our growth is that it be ended in birth, then truly our life is absurd."

Resigned to despair, the one stabbed the darkness with his unseeing eyes and as he clutched his precious life cord to his chest said, "If this is true, and life is absurd, then there really can be no Mother."

"But there is a Mother," protested the other, "Who else gave us nourishment and our world?"

"We get our own nourishment, and our world has always been here. And if there is a Mother, where is she? Have you ever seen her? Does she ever talk to you? No! We invented the Mother because it satisfied a need in us. It make us feel secure and happy."

Thus, while one raved and despaired, the other resigned to birth and placed trust in the hands of the Mother.

Hours stretched into days, and days fell into weeks. And it came time. Both knew their birth was at hand, and both feared what they did not know. As the one was first to be conceived, so he was the first to be born, the other following.

They cried as they were born into the light. And coughed out the fluid and gasped the dry air. And when they were sure they had been born, they opened their eyes seeing for the first time, and found themselves cradled in the warm love of their Mother! They lay open-mouthed and awestruck before the beauty and truth they could not have hoped to have known.

Anonymous

What You Need to Know before You Have Your Baby: Overcoming Common Labor Challenges

Excerpted from, Homebirth – The Essential Guide to Giving Birth Outside of the Hospital, *Sheila Kitzinger 1991. A practical, fact-filled guide for every woman who wants to choose carefully among the alternatives to giving birth in a hospital by the leading female authority on pregnancy and childbirth.*

All that is needed for the majority of labors to go well is a healthy, pregnant woman who has loving support in labor, self-confidence, and attendants with infinite patience. Sadly most women don't have these things, and then even a straightforward labor can become difficult, with rescue maneuvers taking the place of the nurturing that is the basis of good midwifery care.

Women who have their babies in a hospital are more likely to have difficult labors just because they are in a hospital. This is not to say that problems never develop in planned out-of-hospital births, only that they are usually of a kind that can be solved by simple, noninvasive measures. Here are some of the things that can be done to help when difficulties are encountered, so that you, your midwife or doctor, and birth partner can discuss together what action to take.

You Are Overdue

Most babies are not born on the date they are expected. Generally speaking, it is safer for them to be born after the expected date of delivery than preterm. Although with prolonged pregnancy every hour may seem like a week, and each week a month, a baby will usually be born within ten days of the expected date. If you go past ten days, it may be because you had a long menstrual cycle, ovulated later than you thought, and so conceived later, or because the date based on ultrasound that you were given was incorrect. Gestational age based on the known first day of the last menstruation is more accurate than ultrasound. There is a random error of two weeks with ultrasound.

If you go past your due date, it may be reassuring to make a note of fetal movements. A baby who is moving vigorously is fine, although a baby makes fewer whole body movements in the last few weeks of pregnancy, because there is a tighter fit in the uterus. A healthy baby continues to kick, often when you are resting or lying in the bath. A simple way of keeping a movement chart is to select a time of day when your baby is always at its most active and monitor what is happening during that time.

If you find your baby has quieted down, the most likely possibility is that labor is about to start and, in this case, there may be other signs, such as a rush of energy as you feel the nesting instinct and want to clean out cupboards or finish a work project; the need to empty your bladder frequently; a slight looseness of the bowels – like a minor digestive upset; low backache; a feeling that your baby's head is hanging between your legs like a coconut; and more frequent contractions of your uterus. When movements are much reduced and labor does not start, contact your health team.

If all is well, there is no advantage to inducing labor simply because your pregnancy is prolonged. In fact there are disadvantages in inductions, since it greatly increases the chances of a cesarean section. Enjoy these last unanticipated days of pregnancy with special activities which otherwise you might not have the time for, that restaurant you meant to try, the concert you thought you wouldn't be able to go to because the baby would just be born, a day with a friend, a picnic, a trip to an art gallery or museum, a play or film that you can fit in now, or a browse around antique or craft shops. Don't just sit and wait for the first twinges and brood over what seems by now to be an elephant pregnancy. Soon there will be a baby in your arms.

You Think Labor Has Started But It Hasn't

Many women have painful contractions that might be the start of labor in the last few weeks before they actually go into labor. This is prodromal labor, and means that changes are taking place in preparation for labor before dilation starts. It is a sign that contractions are beginning to soften and thin out the cervix and push down the baby's presenting part – the part of the baby nearest your cervix, usually the head. Although tiring, this may reduce the length of time you are in labor.

If this happens to you, it is important to get sleep, perhaps with a special bedtime ritual-soaking in a bath with lavender oil, and then having a hot milk drink with honey, and listening to soothing music as you settle down with a hot water bottle in the small of your back or against your lower abdomen.

Your Water Breaks Before Labor Starts

Ten percent of women have premature rupture of the membranes at term and eight out of ten of these start labor spontaneously within 12 hours, although sometimes a woman has to wait as long as 24 hours before it begins. Premature rupture is more likely when there have been vaginal examinations in the weeks preceding, so that is a good reason for declining such examinations in the last weeks of pregnancy.

When your water breaks, there may be a gush of fluid or a slow trickle. If there is only a dribble of fluid, it is probably the hind waters, the part of the bubble behind the baby's head, that are leaking, and they often reseal themselves after a while. You can ignore it. If there is a gush of fluid, note whether it is clear or stained brown or green. If it is clear, and your baby is already engaged in your pelvis, you do not need to take special action. If it is stained, the baby has emptied its bowels of meconium, a sign that it could be under stress.

You should call your midwife or doctor so that the baby's position can be checked. Often any meconium present is not fresh, which is a sign that the baby was stressed some time ago. If your baby is in a breech position, meconium is squeezed out mechanically as the bottom is pressed down and this is not an indication that the baby is stressed.

An important thing to know when membranes rupture is the position in which your baby is lying. If the baby is head down and the head is low in the pelvis, there is no possibility of the type of emergency occurring when a loop of cord slips down beneath the head. There is a remote chance of this happening if the head is still high, however, or if the baby is lying in a less usual position as in breech or across the uterus. Once your membranes have ruptured, do not put anything inside your vagina or you may introduce infection. There should be no vaginal examinations out of curiosity either. The more vaginal examinations that take place, the greater the risk of infection.

If you wait anxiously for the first contraction, you will be tired out by the time your energy is really needed. So put on a sanitary pad, change it regularly, and go to bed and sleep, do some work around the house or garden, play cards, chess, or Scrabble, listen to music, or watch television. To check that there is no infection, take your temperature every three hours. If there is an infection, you will become slightly feverish, and you should let your caregiver know this. When you empty your bowels, be careful to wipe from front to back, away from your vagina, so that you do not introduce bacteria from your rectum. Don't starve yourself during this wait. You may not want to eat once labor starts, so avoid a long fast now. Have plenty of fluids – fruit juice, tea, or whatever you wish to help replace your amniotic fluid, and keep your energy up with snacks of high carbohydrate food, such as pastas, baked potato, and pancakes with syrup. Some midwives suggest taking supplementary vitamin C to build resistance to infection, 250 mg every few hours.

Prolapsed Cord

A prolapsed cord is an obstetric emergency. It occurs rarely – in 0.3 percent of pregnancies. It happens occasionally in late pregnancy, when membranes rupture prematurely, whether or not a woman intends to have her baby in the hospital. Your midwife will diagnose that the baby's cord is trapped if it can be felt pulsating in your vagina. But sometimes it is too high to feel, and the clue is a marked deceleration in the fetal heart rate, immediately after membrane rupture, when the presenting part is high. Go to the hospital immediately if this happens.

Emergency treatment of cord prolapse is to get into a knee-chest position with your bottom high in the air. Your midwife inserts two clean fingers in your cervix to press the baby's presenting part up and away from the cord. A prolapsed cord is very unlikely to occur during a home birth or in any birthplace where invasive procedures are not practiced. It is usually a consequence of intervention, in particular of rupturing the membranes artificially when the presenting part is very high.

A Long, Slow Labor

It is difficult to time the onset of labor precisely and although some women are suddenly aware that this is IT, far more experience a gentle lead-in to labor. The arbitrary decision made by some obstetricians that labor must not last longer than 12 hours, or that dilation must proceed by I cm per hour, puts the woman under stress and makes her attendants anxious so that they sometimes act unwisely in an attempt to hurry labor along. They may rupture the membranes in order to hasten a slow labor. But if this is done before 4 cm dilation of the cervix it can actually slow down an already slow labor. In a hospital a long, slow labor is often termed failure to progress, (FTP), only because caregivers find the waiting intolerable. Most long labors are simply variations on a theme, and there is an art in adapting to them and not being hassled or discouraged.

If your labor is slow intersperse activity and rest and change your activities frequently. Avoid boredom. Bake a cake for the celebration afterward, soak in a bath, go for a walk, sew or knit – anything rather than lying in bed wondering if there is something wrong because labor is not going faster.

Eat easily digested, smooth foods such as potato puree, soup, mashed banana, ice cream, sorbet, honey sandwiches, or yogurt, and drink plenty of fluids. Raspberry leaf tea has a mild oxytocic action and may help as well.

Move around and keep changing position in order to stimulate uterine activity, and to encourage the baby to descend and rotate with the crown of the head against your cervix. Rock your pelvis, go up and down stairs, and lunge against the wall.

Soak in a bath or have a shower to refresh you and help you to relax.

Empty your bladder every hour and a half to two hours.

A woman in slow labor welcomes quiet, calm reassurance from the attendants. You should not feel under any pressure of time. It is often good to be left alone with your partner.

Explore what happens when you do nipple stimulation or gentle clitoral massage. You can simply get into bed, send everyone away, turn off the light and have a cuddle with your partner for an hour or two.

Start – Stop Labor

Some labors are slow in a different way. They start and then seem to stop. The uterus contracts weakly or ceases to contract for an interval, then starts again, but may have another phase of inactivity. There may be plateaus like this when nothing much seems to be happening. A start-stop labor occurs most commonly when a woman is admitted to a hospital and her previous regular, strong contractions become spasmodic. The cause is anxiety. The uterus is very responsive to anxiety and this is as true for other mammals as for women. Interference can make any animal's labor more difficult. Bring what is bothering you out into the open and have your birth partner or midwife help you deal with it.

There is a physical cause for some start-stop labors. The baby's head can be in an awkward position and become stuck. Your midwife will monitor the fetal heart regularly and assess the situation. When a baby is awkwardly positioned, moving about and rocking and rolling your pelvis may coax the baby into a better position so that labor can progress. And even when the head is a tight fit, and the baby's descent through the pelvis is delayed, the spontaneous movements a woman makes can assist the uterus to ease the baby's head through the cervix and down the birth canal.

A Lull at the End of the First Stage

When the baby's head is high and still above the level of the ischial spines there is often a pause at the very end of the first stage of labor. The uterus rests, and everyone else can rest as well. In hospital, during this pause, the decision is often made to set up a Pitocin drip in order to stimulate the uterus into action. Both in hospital and at home it is wiser to wait for descent and rotation of the head to occur, and at the same time give your body a chance to prepare for the active second stage. Squatting is a good position for initiating contractions and encouraging rotation of the baby's head so that it can press against your pelvic floor muscles. When the head touches nerves in these muscles, the pushing reflex is stimulated, and oxytocin spurts into your bloodstream, causing strong contractions. If you start pushing simply because you are fully dilated and have been told to do so, but do not feel the spontaneous reflex, you can become exhausted with straining, and are likely to push the baby's head down unrotated, with resulting deep transverse arrest, when the baby cannot turn its head to the easiest position for delivery. In most labors this is completely avoidable if a woman is not urged to push too soon and if everyone waits patiently.

Morale Drops

Most women feel that they can't go on and would like to postpone having the baby when they reach the end of the first stage of labor. These feelings are a sign of progress; for this is transition, the bridge between the first and second stage. If there comes a time in labor when you are discouraged, you need change:

Change your position or the kind of movements you are making.

Find a change of scene. Move to another room or go outside.

Try changing the rhythm of your breathing.

Ask for a change in the kind of touch you are receiving.

Have someone new come in and stay with you.

If you have been in semi-darkness, now light a lot of candles or turn the lights up. If the room is bright, draw the curtains or dim the lights.

If you have music in the background, change the tape.

If you have had your eyes closed during contractions, open them now.

Perhaps you have been silent during contractions. Now open up and make low sounds that go right down into your pelvis.

Make an opportunity to freshen up. Splash your face with cold water. Have a bath or shower. Suck cracked ice.

Pep up your energy with a glucose drink or spoonfuls of honey.

Worries about the Fetal Heart Rate

The important thing about the baby's heart rate is that, if it slows a lot as contractions reach their peak, it should pick up again about 15 seconds after the end of a contraction. If it does this, the baby is receiving plenty of oxygen. Continue to change your position and change your breathing while monitoring the heart beat as this can often remedy matters.

You Are Hyperventilating

Hyperventilation is the result of breathing in and out fast and furiously. It often happens at the end of the first stage, when contractions are coming at two minute intervals. The woman breathes too heavily and allows no time for the slight pauses that come naturally between inspiration and expiration. You can avoid hyperventilating by keeping your shoulders and throat relaxed, by focusing on the idea of relaxing a little more with each breath out, and by letting your breathing flow rhythmically. Your helpers can breathe with you so that you do not feel so alone.

You Become Very Tired

Labor is an intense, energy consuming activity, and may be the most strenuous work you have ever done. A woman often feels as if she is on a treadmill of contractions. Have a drink that will adjust your body's electrolyte balance. "Labor Aid" can be made by mixing together I quart water, 1/3 cup honey. 1/3 cup lemon juice, 1/2 teaspoon salt, 1/4 teaspoon baking powder and two crushed calcium tablets. Eat something that does not need much chewing and can just slip down. Do not fight the pain. Go right into it instead. Whatever happens during contractions make sure that you are resting completely in each interval between. Remember that you are having a baby. Extra encouragement at this time may give you a fresh heart.

You Have a Pushing Urge before Being Fully Dialated

A woman may have the desire to push before her cervix is fully open. Pushing hard against an incompletely dilated cervix can make it puffy and swollen so that it actually closes a little. If you want to push and are not yet 10 cm dilated, you may find the following suggestions helpful: Continue breathing. Do not hold your breath, when the longing to push comes, give two quick breaths out followed by one slow breath out, so that there is a steady rhythm of pant, pant, blow, breath in. It sometimes helps if your birth partner holds up a finger in front of your mouth so that you can direct each blow onto it. As soon as the urge leaves you, breathe fully and easily again. If you are in an upright position, this is the time to change it and lie down on your side or be on all fours. If you have to push, do so with an open mouth and breathing out. Let your uterus do the work while you open up.

You Get No Pushing Urge

A women can have a baby without deliberately pushing it out. Her uterus sees to that. Until there is an irresistible urge to push, it is sensible to avoid pushing by continuing to breathe. There is no need to hold your breath at all. In this way, all the tissues have a chance to fan out smoothly before the ball of the baby's head eases through, with no damage to ligaments, muscles, or skin. Go with your body. When you are free to follow your uterus, the pushing rhythm which it dictates may vary with different contractions. Some pushes are short and others long. Sometimes there is only one push with a contraction, at other times four or five. Even if you feel unsure about what to do, your body knows how to give birth.

Meconium Is Passed

The bowels of a mature fetus contain meconium, and if the baby is under stress this meconium is expelled in the amniotic fluid. The presence of meconium is a sign of maturity, but it can also mean that the baby is stressed. If the baby inhales meconium, there is a chance that respiratory tract infection can develop. If you are nowhere near birth when meconium is passed, your attendants will probably suggest that you transfer to the hospital so that a pediatrician can be ready to resuscitate if necessary.

If the baby is about to be born and fresh meconium is passed, your midwife or doctor will simply have a mucus extractor ready to suck out meconium gently – even before the baby's body is born, and before the chest has expanded to take the first breath. It will be easier to do this if you stand with your knees bent or are on all fours. Breathe the baby out gently, rather than pushing, and there will be time for your caregiver to suction out every bit of meconium.

The Baby Is Coming Very Fast

When the second stage is rapid and it looks as if the baby will pop out like a champagne cork, there are several things you can do to slow down the pace and make birth gentler: Adopt an all fours position, or lie on your side, so that your midwife or doctor can guard your perineum with a hand. Do not squat or stand. Breath the baby out. Guide your baby down with your breathing. Avoid pushing. If you have to push, breathe again as soon as possible. Release your pelvic floor muscles and relax your perineum by opening your mouth and dropping your jaw. If you want to make noises, moo, bellow, groan, or give deep sighs – resonant sounds that go right down into your pelvis. Do not scream or yelp as that will make you tighten up. Listen closely and be guided by your midwife or doctor.

The Baby Is a Surprise Breech

Occasionally labor is going well and the birth attendants see something emerging that looks like a bald head, and realize, perhaps after meconium is squeezed out, that it is the baby's bottom. This is an undiagnosed breech. Breech labor is like any other labor up to the point when the baby's body slips out. What may then happen is that the head gets stuck. A breech baby should always be delivered gently to avoid injury to the spinal cord, arms and neck.

Left to itself, the baby's body uncurls, the uterus keeps the head flexed, and one or both legs drop out, followed by the body and then the head. In a series of 89 breech births delivered by midwives in New Jersey there was not a single case of extended arms and all the babies were fine. Never forcibly pull the legs in a breech birth as this will cause the baby to become stuck when the arms extend.

If you have a surprise breech, adopt a supported, upright position, legs wide apart and knees bent, in order to give the baby's head the most space and to enable gravity to help it slip through. The worst possible position for a breech delivery is lying on your back with legs raised in stirrups. In that position your sacrum and coccyx are pressed up and the dimensions of your pelvic cavity and outlet are reduced. If you squat, you gain an extra centimeter across your pelvic cavity and two centimeters from front to back.

Once you have adopted a half-standing, half-squatting position, leaning on your birth partner in front of you, your midwife or doctor should be positioned behind you, and should simply wait and watch until the baby's body is completely born. The only intervention that may be necessary is to press gently behind the baby's knees if the feet are up over the shoulders. This will stimulate the baby to bend the knees so that they come down. When the legs are extended, they splint the spine, so that it is more difficult for the baby to take the curve of the birth canal.

As you bend your knees and go into a deep squat, holding on to your birth partner, the baby's body will slip out. The cord may slide down too and if it is wrapped tightly around the baby, your midwife or doctor will carefully unloop it, but only very gently, or it may go into spasm. You may feel a confusing, intermittent pushing urge. Avoid pushing if you can until the head is ready to emerge. Let the baby be born by uterine activity alone. This will enable everything to open up and your tissues to spread wide. As soon as the whole body is born, drop forward, legs still wide apart and knees bent, leaning over some furniture, or your birth partner so that your back is almost horizontal. This tilts your pelvis so that the baby's nose and mouth are visible, and whoever is catching the baby can aspirate the nose and mouth with a mucus extractor before the head is fully born. A breech baby often begins to breathe once its chest is born, and may inhale mucus from your birth canal. The mucus can block the nasal passages and although most babies are clever at sneezing out anything that is irritating, in this case manual aspiration is a wise precaution.

Shoulder Dystocia

When a baby is head down, sometimes a big head is born, and then there is a delay in the delivery of the shoulders. Very rarely the shoulders really are stuck; this is known as shoulder dystocia. If your baby's head is born and then nothing happens, move! Movement itself often releases the shoulders. You may choose a hands and knees position and when the next contraction comes, push hard as your helper applies gentle downward traction to the head. The baby sometimes falls out. Another very good position is to stand with your knees as wide apart as possible. If your baby still does not budge, your helper will reach in with two fingers and find the baby's posterior armpit, the one nearest, and either pull the shoulder forward or pull down the arm. A fourteen pound baby can be delivered this way with no need at all for an episiotomy.

Twins

If you have undiagnosed twins or labor with diagnosed twins proceeds too quickly to risk getting to a hospital: Warm the room and fill hot-water bottles so that the babies will not become cold. Small babies are quickly chilled. Stay calm and peaceful, even though this is very exciting. Breathe with a gentle expiration as slowly as you comfortably can. You are breathing for your babies.

Once in the second stage, take it as gently as possible and avoid both hyperventilating and prolonged breath holding. Your first baby may cope well with these, but the second baby needs good oxygenation for a while longer. Choose any position that is comfortable for you – preferably an upright one (standing, squatting, kneeling, or half-kneeling, half-squatting). If labor is progressing very rapidly, get on all fours. When the first baby is born, put her to your breast. The sucking will stimulate further contractions to bring the next baby to birth.

The Baby Who Is Slow To Breathe

Babies are enormously adaptable. Then can manage with very little oxygen for much longer than an adult. Some babies start to breathe as soon as their heads are born. Most take a few seconds to get going. When the cord is not clamped immediately, and it is pulsating, the baby is still receiving a little oxygenated blood straight into her bloodstream. There need be no rush to force her to breathe.

When a baby is born with the mother in an upright position mucus drains naturally from the mouth and nose. Newborn babies often sneeze mucus out very effectively too. If a baby needs help to breathe, the first thing to do is to make sure that the airways are clear. She can be placed on her front with the head lower than the hips, so that mucus drains out, while you gently massage her back. If your baby has had a long and difficult transition she will need warmth most of all. Otherwise she uses up a great deal of energy trying to maintain body heat. Most heat loss is from the head, so she should be wrapped in warmed flannel blankets and her head covered.

There can be a spiritual element in helping a baby to life. If your baby is just flickering and is starting, but not quite managing, to breathe, it helps to talk to your baby, to say "Hello, baby," "Come on love, come on!" or "You're beautiful!" The result may be that the lungs open wider, breaths are deeper, and respiration is more regular. In intensive care nurseries, where babies are being monitored very carefully, oxygen levels often rise when a baby is stroked and when the mother speaks to her baby.

You Have Heavy Bleeding

During your pregnancy a steady flow of blood or continual spotting can mean that the placenta is starting to peel away from the lining of the uterus (placental abruption) or that it is in front of the baby's head (placenta previa). Let your midwife or doctor know what is happening. They will probably get you into hospital as quickly as they can, as an examination should only be done once everything has been set up for cesarean section, should it be necessary.

After your labor and delivery your uterus continues to contract, although you may not be aware of it. The placenta cannot contract, so it peels away from the lining of the uterus, usually within half an hour of the birth, and slips down into your vagina. When this happens and the placenta is ready to be expelled, some bright red blood appears and the cord lengthens. Until the placenta separates from the uterine wall there is no bleeding and even though the placenta may remain in the uterus for a long time, this is not dangerous. Your midwife or doctor may gently press in above your pubic bone and push upward toward your navel to see if the cord moves up as the uterus is tipped upward. If it does, the placenta is still attached and no one should pull on the cord or it may cause bleeding.

The best way to assist your body in detaching from your placenta is to stand upright and blow into an empty bottle. As air is exhaled, the abdominal press comes into play so that the mother's abdominal muscles press on her fundus and propel the placenta down. Tugging or pulling on the cord can cause hemorrhage and should never be done. A postpartum hemorrhage happens when a placenta does not peel away completely, and blood seeps from gaping sinuses in the muscle wall of the uterus. Left to itself the uterus will clamp down uniformly and will sheer off the placenta in one smooth sweep, but if poked and prodded may only release in certain sections.

Gently massaging your uterus and nipple stimulation will keep your uterus firm and contracting to assist in the expulsion of your placenta. When the placenta is delivered, your midwife or doctor will check your pulse and blood pressure and may ask you to continue massaging the uterus to keep it well contracted.

Home Birth Advantages

A carefully planned and lovingly conducted home birth, in which the rhythms of nature are respected and the woman is nurtured by attendants who have the knowledge and understanding to support the spontaneous unfolding of life, is the safest kind of birth there is, and the most deeply satisfying for everyone involved.

Babytime

Around this time you will have increasing prelabor start-stop contractions, you may lose your mucous plug, your water may leak or gush, you may feel your baby's head drop lower in your pelvis giving you more room to breath and you will begin to feel impatient and excited about your baby's impending arrival. None of these signs mean that your labor has actually started. Keep in close contact with your health team during this period letting them know of each new development as it happens. A first-time mother can labor for days or many hours before going into the delivery stage and moving too quickly to the hospital can frustrate everyone. This is where your professional labor support person can be an invaluable asset to you as she will come to your home when your labor actually begins and can time your departure to the hospital or birthing clinic closely if you will be leaving your home.

Go for a massage.

Find a family member to walk with.

Work in your garden.

Go swimming.

Take long naps.

Talk to you baby in the womb. Your baby hears loud noises very well at this stage so explain shower or bath noises, the vacuum cleaner noise, the doorbell or buzzer, telephone ringing and other sounds.

Babies in utero usually sleep during the day as you rock them to sleep with your movements. If kicking is really getting to you, going for a walk can rock your baby back to sleep giving both of you a break.

Eat and drink well to prepare your body and your baby for the upcoming delivery.

Relax and remember that babies are not machines, a normal delivery is between 38 and 42 weeks and longer. Remind your doctor of this should he mention inductions. The more natural your birth, the easier labor and delivery will be for both you and baby. As soon as your doctor or health team intervenes it can set up a chain of events from which there is no turning back. As long as you feel your baby and you are in good health, delay any interventions until you go into natural labor. Watching and waiting at this time can make your labor faster and easier for both you and your baby. If you are feeling pressure from your team to have your baby by a certain date, get a second and third opinion. Don't buy into the myth that after 40 weeks your placenta won't sufficiently nurture your baby.

This is the best time for shopping, finishing the baby's room, and getting organized for your baby's arrival.

10

Your Partner's Role in Childbirth

More men than ever, to their credit, are taking an active, involved interest in the birth of their children. Your partner wants to be involved by becoming a part of the decision process. Your partner has a critical role to play as your advocate. Write your birth plan together so that everyone is aware of what is important to you.

Your partner is not labor support unless your partner has personally birthed a baby. Fathers are "birthing" as well and this situation is just as new to him. Hiring professional labor support, such as a doula or midwife, during your first birth is an excellent investment and can take the pressure off your partner. Your partner and family can then provide the emotional support that is just as necessary.

Make sure you have a partner. Your partner does not have to be your mate; anyone you love and trust will do.

Your birth partner, whether your mate, your midwife, your mother, your sister, your best friend, your next door neighbor, or a combination of the above will give you the emotional support necessary to see you through.

The support of your partner will often depend on the preparation they have received in prenatal classes. The Bradley Method of Husband-Coached Childbirth classes focus on giving your partner adequate knowledge so that they can become your advocate in labor. The Childbirth Resource Directory in this guide will refer you to other equally informative prenatal classes in Canada and the United States.

You may wish to have people you know come in shifts if you have a large family or many supportive friends. Having a few people come in on and off during your labor can help you to keep your sense of humor when you need it most. Birth is a great celebration of life and touches deeply all involved in the process.

Here are a few ideas of what your partner can do for you during labor and delivery:

- Ask your partner to make sure that you have plenty of water, juices and tea to drink.
- Have your partner remind you to breath slowly and deeply.
- Have your partner remind you to urinate every hour to make more room for your baby's descent.
- Have your partner massage your lower back, neck and shoulders. Current research shows that as you become more relaxed during labor your pain decreases. Thus a warm bath or shower, a gentle massage, a shoulder to lean against, a gentle hug, encouraging words and a hand to grip will aid greatly in naturally reducing pain during labor.
- Let your partner know before labor how much you love him. Warn him that sometimes women say things during labor that they don't mean. Let him know not to take anything personally.
- Your partner is your cheering section. Even whispered words of encouragement can help see you through to the end.
- Be clear in telling your partner what you need during labor, don't assume or expect your partner will know what you want during each stage.
- Walk around the hospital as much as possible during your labor and use your partner to lean on during contractions. Having someone to lean on when you are standing during a contraction seems to shorten the length of the contraction.
- Your partner should encourage you to change positions whenever you can. Moving into a new position, standing, walking, resting on the left side, kneeling, moving to the bath, climbing stairs, squatting, and leaning over furniture helps your body and your baby to work more efficiently.
- During delivery, have your partner hold the mirror so that you can see your baby's head crown to more easily control the pushing stage.
- Have your partner or professional labor support use the warmed oil you have brought to massage your perineum and your baby's head to ease delivery.
- Have your partner or professional labor support provide gentle counter pressure to your baby's head and your perineum allowing for a safe, controlled delivery of the shoulders and chest.
- Have your partner or midwife bring your baby to your breast for the first time as quickly as possible after birth. Breastfeeding immediately after birth releases hormones to help your body birth the placenta and to stop excessive bleeding.
- Standing while blowing into an empty bottle will also help your body to more efficiently release your placenta. Never let anyone pull on the cord of your placenta. This can cause bleeding. There is no hurry for the

placenta to be delivered or removed.

- Have your partner be in charge of cutting your baby's umbilical cord. Some couples tie the umbilical cord with a cotton cord instead using of a plastic clamp. The umbilical cord seems to heal faster with less chance of infection when cotton is used.
- Ask your partner to closely examine the placenta. Look at your placenta as well to assure yourself that the entire placenta has been delivered.
- Have your partner take your baby's first pictures using the disposable instant flash camera you have brought along. Disposable cameras are easy to work, always ready and allow you to be sure you will capture the first precious moments of your baby's life.
- Invite your professional labor support person to take your first family photograph. You will always treasure these photographs and your baby will too.

What You Need to Know before You Have Your Baby: Professional Labor Support – What To Expect
Excerpted from Mothering the Mother – How A Doula Can Help You Have a Shorter, Easier, and Healthier Birth *Marshall H Klaus, M.D., John H. Kennell, M.D., and Phyllis H. Klaus, M.Ed.,C.S.W. 1993*

Early First Stage of Childbirth – Prelabor & Labor
The efforts of the doula or childbirth assistant during the first stage, when the cervix thins and opens, should be geared toward helping the mother have a relaxed body and a mind at peace. This allows the mother's contracting uterus to open her cervix while she conserves her energy for pushing. You can help her with the following measures:

Have the mother stay home as long as possible. Options for comfort are much greater at home. Going into the hospital will not make things happen faster, and labor may even slow down in a strange environment.

During this early time in labor a woman can gradually get used to the feeling of contractions. Later, as contractions become more intense, they will hurt. This pain is a normal part of the birthing process. Remind the mother that there is a purpose for the pain; it is a sign of the work her body is doing to thin and open her cervix. To help her accept and cope with the pain, you can remind her that she is not in this alone.

It is essential for a woman to take nourishment in the form of fluids or easily digestible proteins and carbohydrates. A dehydrated or starved body cannot labor as effectively as a well nourished one. Also, the baby continues to be totally dependent on her for nourishment throughout labor. Suggest that she eat a good meal early in labor, and have her continue to drink plenty of liquids and avoid high-fat foods and concentrated sweets. The mother might wish to try juice, fruit, yogurt, whole-wheat bread or crackers, nourishing soup, and other foods that appeal to her. As labor progresses, she may not feel like eating, but encourage her to drink. Labor is hard work, and she will need lots of fluid to meet her body's needs. If fruit juices do not appeal to her, suggest non-caffeinated soft drinks, which will give her the energy she needs without making her feel jittery. Nausea is normal for some women in labor and is not the result of drinking or eating.

Suggest a warm bath to help her stay more comfortable and relaxed. Fill the tub as high as possible. Have her kneel in the tub or lie back against pillows. Keep a comfortably hot, wet towel over her belly and groin during contractions. She might want a cool drink and a cool cloth for her head. Be sure to give this a try, especially at times in labor when the mother feels that nothing will help.

Have the mother walk. Walking tends to shorten labor, reduce the need for pain-relieving drugs, decrease fetal heart-rate abnormalities, and improve the baby's condition during labor and birth. A doula and other support people may need to keep encouraging the mother strongly to walk.

Women in labor should change positions often-at least every thirty to sixty minutes. This can help to avoid or correct fetal distress, as well as speed labor. Positions such as standing, squatting, and kneeling while leaning forward are excellent. They can increase uterine activity, shorten labor by helping the cervix dilate more efficiently, and reduce discomfort. Other good positions for labor include sitting, lying on the side, and being up on the hands and knees. Use lots of pillows to help the mother feel comfortable. She should not lie flat on her back because this can cause a drop in her blood pressure and a decreased blood flow and therefore decreased oxygen to her baby. Laboring women should urinate every hour. A full bladder can inhibit uterine activity and be an obstacle to the baby's birth.

Late First Stage of Childbirth – Transition Period

During the late first stage of labor, most women strongly need other people, their support people, to help them cope with and accept the intense contractions that are normal for this time in labor. Labor is truly easier when a woman has people to encourage and reassure her during this time. If she is going to a hospital or birth center for her baby's birth, the best time to make the trip is usually late in the first stage. Whether at home or in the hospital or birth center, the following measures will continue to be helpful.

Have the mother continue with warm baths or showers, hot towels, position changes, walking, nourishment, and frequent urination. Try other comfort measures such as cold compresses, pressure on her back, pelvic rocking, massages or stroking. Let the mother use extra pillows, a bean bag, or you or the father to lean against for added comfort. What feels good often changes as labor progresses, so remember to try again with comfort measures that may not have been helpful earlier.

This is an intense time. The mother may need to maintain contact with you through every contraction. You can talk and breathe her through contractions, use a loving touch, and maintain eye contact. Then help her rest, relax and refresh herself between contractions. Visualizations and imagery are also extremely useful to help the mother work through the contractions.

Ask the mother to show or tell you not only how and where to touch her but also what feels good and what does not.

Help the mother stay upright and walking as long as possible. Alternate periods of activity and rest as needed. She may need a lot of encouragement to change position, walk, or urinate. Remember, these activities will help her labor progress normally.

Many women experience a time in labor when they are in a lot of pain and cannot get comfortable. If the mother experiences these feelings, help her concentrate on releasing tension and yielding to the intense contractions. Emotional support and focus on relaxation, in spite of the intensity of the contractions, will get her through this difficult time. Reassure her that she can do it. Have her deal with her contractions one at a time and not think about how long it has been or how long it will be.

The Second Stage of Childbirth – Delivery

The doula's efforts and those of the father during the second stage, when the cervix is completely open and the mother pushes her baby out, should be geared not only toward helping her cooperate with her body but also toward providing a calm, peaceful atmosphere into which her new child will be born.

During this stage you, the doula, can help in the following ways: There is nothing magical about a woman being at ten centimeters, or completely dilated. Some women feel an urge to push before ten centimeters, and others feel it considerably after this point.

If the mother does not feel an urge to push, try getting her into a gravity assisted upright position and continue to breathe with her through contractions. Walking, squatting, or sitting on the toilet often helps at this time. Remind the mother to be patient, relax, and wait for a pushing urge to develop as her baby moves farther down her birth canal. Waiting until the urge to push develops allows her to coordinate her pushing efforts with those of her uterus. If her physician or midwife feels it is necessary to birth her baby quickly, she or he will direct her on how and when to push.

Have the woman urinate before she begins pushing.

Any positions used for labor can also be used for pushing and for the baby's birth. Each position has advantages and disadvantages. A mother who has practiced during pregnancy and experimented during labor may know the most comfortable and effective positions. Help her change positions at least every half hour if she has a long or difficult second stage. Upright positions that use gravity may be helpful. Squatting uses gravity and allows maximum opening of the pelvic outlet. Standing sometimes helps if the baby is still high in the pelvis. Sitting on the toilet is excellent for opening up and releasing the whole pelvic area. Lying on one side can be helpful in slowing a quick descent, but less helpful if the baby is coming slowly. Upright positions can aggravate hemorrhoids; lying on the side does not. All fours positions do not use gravity, but they do take pressure off the back and allow spreading of the hips and pelvic bones. Both all fours and squatting positions are good for a large or posterior baby.

Avoid letting the mother lie flat on her back. If she is semi-reclining, you or the father can sit behind her to prop her up, or you can use pillows or raise the head of the birthing bed or delivery table so that she is not lying flat.

The mother will need frequent assurance that the intense and painful sensations she may feel – backache, nausea, hot flashes, trembling legs, spreading sensations in the pelvis, intense pressure on the rectum, an urge to empty the bowels, involuntary bearing down, intense pressure as the baby descends through the birth canal, or burning and stretching sensations as the vaginal outlet opens to accommodate her baby – are normal and that she can stretch and open enough to give birth to her baby.

Remind her to work with her body – let her body tell her what to do to get her baby out. She can bear down, push, when, how, and however long her body demands that. Encourage her to ease up on pushing if it hurts or if burning sensations occur. She may want to see and touch her baby's head as it emerges from her body. This contact may renew her spirits and energy, and help her focus on bringing her baby out.

When pushing, she might at times breathe out, make noise, or hold her breath. Many women have found that certain noises like grunts and moaning sounds help them give birth to their babies. Help her not to be inhibited about making sounds which is a natural part of the birthing process for many women, and she will find what works for her if she goes ahead and tries it. Many women find that releasing sound opens the throat and subsequently the birth canal. Have her avoid prolonged breath holding.

During a long second stage, a woman needs nourishment to keep up or restore her energy level. Spoonfuls of honey or drinks sweetened with honey or juice will provide a quick source of energy.

You can encourage her to release and open for the birth. If you watch her mouth, shoulders, and legs for signs of tension, you can help her release these areas. She may be so intently focused on the work of giving birth that she does not hear what others are saying. You can help by keeping the mother informed of what is happening and conveying instructions from the health team or midwife.

Keep the atmosphere calm and peaceful, so that the mother and father can enjoy the end of labor and the new life they have brought forth.

11

Secrets to Having a
Faster and Easier Labor and Delivery

Labor

- Labor contractions are very similar to your period cramps when they begin.
- Your labor can take days or hours.
- Hire professional labor support to assist you and your partner.
- Practice, prepack and preplan for this special day.
- Remain as "relaxed" and as focused as you can.
- Work with your body.
- Trust yourself and your body to deliver your baby safely.
- Breath deeply throughout your labor. Your baby and your body need all the oxygen you can give now. See yourself giving your baby extra energy with each long slow breath you take. Work together with your baby and see your baby beginning to descend out through your birth canal as your cervix slowly and easily expands to allow your baby's head through.
- Remember that each contraction brings you one step closer to your baby's birth.
- Visualize your cervix dilating as two great oak doors sliding slowly open. Or as a rose gently opening its petals.
- Don't be embarrassed during your labor, the doctors, nurses and midwives have seen it all. Modesty can inhibit your labor, save it for after your baby is born.
- If anyone is upsetting you with their presence during your labor feel free to ask them to leave the room.
- Focus on having your body work with the contraction. Feel your cervix opening with each contraction and visualize your baby moving further down towards the opening. Working with the contractions and

surrendering to them will help to move your baby along.

- Don't waste your energy and your body's oxygen supply by screaming or fighting. Your energy is the fuel needed to propel your baby into the world. Anything else is counterproductive.
- Grunting or groaning at a low level can help when you feel intense pain.
- Your mind can be your most powerful resource during childbirth. Use your mind to focus inward on the rhythm of your labor.
- Take an epidural only as a last resort. An epidural can cause serious side effects to you and your baby, as well as slow down the most critical part of your labor. The greatest stress on your body happens during the transition stage of your labor and an epidural will not work at this stage.
- During labor walk and stand as much as possible. Gravity will help your baby through your birth canal. Placing your arms around your partner and slightly suspending your weight on him can lessen the pain of a contraction and will assist in moving your baby down.
- Moving about during your labor will help you to feel more in control and will make your labor faster and easier. Change your position as often as you can. Go from sitting or standing, to sitting on the toilet, to leaning forward on the bed, to a squatting position on the floor, to a rocking chair, walking up or down stairs, back to the shower and back again to the toilet.
- If you are experiencing back labor moving to all fours either on the floor or bed will help your team to work on massaging your back to ease muscle spasms. A warm shower or bath is also an excellent way to reduce the pain of back labor. Counter pressure applied during contractions to your tailbone can help as well.
- Holding your partner's hand can give you the extra strength you need at this time.
- Try putting your focus on a favorite photograph or favorite song.
- Fighting and tensing up will increase the pain. Accepting, relaxing and working with the wave-like contractions will decrease the pain.

Delivery

- Delivery is very similar to having a bowel movement.
- Delivery can last hours or minutes.
- Reach down and feel your baby's head with your hand to connect with the miracle of your baby's birth.
- Touching your baby as the head crowns can also help you to focus your energy.
- Squatting opens your pelvic area by 30% and speeds delivery.
- Sitting on the toilet is a good birthing position as it is one of the best

ways to isolate the muscles you will use to push your baby out.

- A squatting bar on the bed is also an excellent birthing position as it allows you total control and you can view your baby's head crowning in a mirror.
- Plan to have your perineum massaged with warm oil as this will stretch the muscles and help your baby to slide out easily. Warm water compresses can also help the perineum to stretch without tearing.
- Squatting for the final stages of delivery can help you to retain some sense of privacy.
- When pushing, use your vaginal muscles to keep your baby from moving back from the birth opening at the end of the contraction. Short pushes are much more effective than long strenuous pushing. Continue even breathing. Short pants with your pushes can be very effective. Watching in the mirror will help you to isolate these muscles more easily.
- When asked to stop pushing, make sure you do. An extra push at this time can cause you to tear. The easiest delivery for both baby and mother is a slow, controlled delivery. Remind yourself that the pain will end the moment your baby is fully born.
- The "ring of fire", as your baby's head crowns fully, is the most painful part of childbirth. Luckily nature is kind and with an unmedicated birth crowning rarely lasts for longer than three pushes.
- Proper perineum support from your professional labor coach will also help to create a slow, controlled delivery.
- If you are told to stop pushing and are having difficulty with it, switch to a kneeling position and you will have more control.
- Should any difficulty arise during your delivery your best position will be in a supported squat, allowing your baby every bit of extra room needed for a faster delivery.
- Put your baby immediately to your breast, within a few minutes after birth. In your baby's first hour the natural instinct to suck is the strongest. Most babies know how to suck, just make your breast available. Do not let your baby suck on just your nipple, make sure your baby's mouth is open wide enough to allow the entire aeriola, or most of it, as well as your nipple into the mouth as this is the correct latch. Breastfeed as long as you feel comfortable on both sides. Always express some drops of milk or colostrum and let air dry on your nipple after feeding to heal any nipple soreness. Do not take breastfeeding advice from anyone who has never breastfed. Professional female assistance is needed for all matters concerning breastfeeding.
- As you are breastfeeding your baby for the first time, oxytocin will be naturally released throughout your system to help your body to slow

down blood loss and to eject your placenta. You will feel more contractions now as your body works to expel your placenta.

- Stand and blow into an empty bottle to assist your body to expel your placenta.
- Do not allow anyone to tug or pull on the cord for your placenta. Allow your body to slowly release your placenta. There is no reason for this stage to be rushed.
- Have your partner check your placenta once it is delivered for any missing pieces or sections. This is the most critical aspect of having a safe birth and delivery. If any of the placenta is left inside of your womb, it can lead to you being unable to bear any more children. Ask to see the placenta yourself to assure yourself that it has been completely delivered.
- Have your partner feed you right after delivery and it will bring your energy up again.
- Plan to Kangaroo Care your baby for the first week. Keeping your baby in bed with you and constantly at your side during this time will increase your baby's immunity and help you to feel more attached to your baby.
- If you are in a hospital and you feel well you may want to take your baby home with you in the next few hours and have your health team come into your home to check on you and your new baby in the days to follow. If you choose a free-standing birth clinic you will naturally be leaving with your baby in two or three hours with the midwives coming to your home for each of the next three days.

12
Breastfeeding Tips

Begin to breastfeed your baby immediately after birth. The reflex to suck is the strongest during the first hour after birth. Let your birthing team know of your intention to breastfeed immediately after birth.

How to Breastfeed Your Baby

1. Select a peaceful setting.
2. Find a comfortable position using good arm and back support.
3. Do not hurry. Remember you have all the time in the world.
4. Pick up your baby before your baby gets fretful.
5. Drop your shoulders, breath out and relax as you put your baby to your breast.
6. Make sure that your baby is latched onto your areola, not just your nipple. Your baby's nose and chin should be touching your breast. This is the correct latch.
7. Remain quiet, speaking to your baby after the feeding.
8. Do not interrupt your feeding time with your baby.
9. Enjoy the time you have together. Make it peaceful and relaxing for you both.
10. Drain your first breast completely before starting on the next. Smaller babies may want to take a short rest in between breasts. In the first month feed your baby whenever your baby cries for as long as your baby needs to feed. This will adjust your supply to your baby's exact needs. Put your watch and schedules away and relax.
    - Breastfeeding is an acquired skill for both baby and mom, just like playing the piano or driving a car. Make sure you have professional breastfeeding support for the first day and week. If you are in a hospital, ask for the lactation consultant to see you immediately. Nurses are too busy to take this special time for every mother and often do not have professional training in breastfeeding.

- It can take four to six weeks to get mom and baby used to breastfeeding. Your body is going through a tremendous adjustment and so is your baby. Make a commitment to stick to it. Don't give up if you become faced with a problem. There are times during this period when it will seem impossible, but once it all comes together breastfeeding will become second nature to you both. As you both become more skilled each feeding will take a shorter duration, you will be producing a greater volume of milk and your baby will need fewer feedings.
- Be persistent and patient.
- If you have not yet attended a breastfeeding clinic or meeting, find a Lactation Consultant and arrange for her to come out to talk to you. She will quickly assist you in answering any questions and taking care of any problems you may have while they are small.
- Help your partner to become comfortable with your breastfeeding by answering any questions he may have and letting him know how much easier, healthier, and inexpensive breastfeeding will be for your family. Talk about what he can do to nurture and love your baby so that he feels included. Let him know that you plan to express your milk and create a milk bank so that he can experience feeding baby as well.
- Do not let anyone in the hospital or at home feed your baby water. Water will reduce your baby's desire to suck as your baby's stomach will feel full. Make sure everyone who comes in contact with your baby realizes you are breastfeeding and that no one is to feed your baby but you.
- Feed your baby as often as possible in the first few hours after birth. Most babies will then sleep for a solid twenty-four hour period in the first day and night and you will want to give your baby the assurance and warmth of your breasts and heartbeat and to insure that your baby gets as much colostrum as possible. Practice makes perfect in every case of breastfeeding for both mother and baby.
- Your baby's stomach is the size of your baby's closed hand at birth and for the first month your baby will need to breastfeed frequently.
- Breastfeeding is extremely soothing to your baby. Toddlers say breastmilk tastes better than ice cream, one more fact owing to its great popularity with babies.
- If you and your baby are having any difficulties in the hospital use one of their electric breast pumps and have your baby cup fed, syringe fed, or finger tube fed with your breastmilk until you work these problems out. This is especially important for premature babies. Premature babies have their own unique breastfeeding challenges and a quick conversation with a breastfeeding consultant will speed both of you on your way. Breastfeeding and Kangaroo Care for your premature infant can help to

avoid many of the difficulties a premature baby has with adjusting to its new world.

- Let everyone know you plan to work through any difficulties.
- Keep pacifiers, soothers and bottles away from your breastfed baby.
- Leave your top and bra off as much as possible for the first two weeks to facilitate ease of breastfeeding, to air dry nipples and to increase bonding with your baby.
- Always express a few drops of breast milk and let the drops dry naturally on your nipple after each feeding. The milk will sterilize and heal any lacerations on your nipples.
- If you find your baby is choking due to the volume of milk and the speed of your letdown reflex make sure your baby is breastfeeding in a sitting up position. If you lean back in your chair you will slow the flow of your milk.
- After each feeding, make sure to remove any excess air by burping your baby. One way is to hold your baby upright on your lap while putting one hand under your baby's neck and head. Use your other hand to press or pat firmly on your baby's back. You can also put your baby over your shoulder or lean your baby across your knees.

Correct Latch

Almost all breastfeeding difficulties are caused by your baby not being correctly latched onto your breast.

1. Tickle the cheek.
2. Wait for a wide open mouth and bring your baby's head toward your breast.
3. Latch on with your baby taking all of your nipple and most or all of your areola surrounding your nipple. Your nipple should be far back into your baby's mouth. Your baby's nose and chin should be touching your breast.
4. If you wish to hold your breast while latching on make sure your hand is well back from the nipple.

Positioning

Sit your baby up to breastfeed as soon as possible to reduce the stress on your arms and shoulders. Your baby will also enjoy sitting to breastfeed as this will reduce choking and makes swallowing much easier. You can feel how difficult it is to swallow when you are lying flat on your back and how much easier it is to swallow when you are in an upright or semi-upright position.

Experiment with new positions as much as possible. Be creative. Be comfortable. If your breasts are smaller consider investing in a breastfeeding pillow. This is a curved pillow that fits around your waist and helps to hold your baby closer to your nipple; the breastfeeding pillow will ease shoulder and neck pain as well.

Different positions include the cradle hold as described above, the football hold is good for c-section recovery as you hold your baby beside you with her legs up and there is no pressure on your surgery site. If you wish to feed your baby lying down make sure your baby's head is raised higher than the body using a small pillow or your arm to raise your baby's head up.

You can even breastfeed your baby upside down, with your baby's feet towards your head as you are lying down. This is a good position to use if you have a blockage in your breast duct.

Engorgement

Engorgement can happen three to five days after your baby is born or later. This can be the most painful part of breastfeeding and luckily engorgement lasts for only a few days. This is a great time to express and save your extra milk by collecting and freezing. When your milk comes in your breasts will feel hot, you may have a fever and you will probably feel miserable. You can achieve quick relief with a bag of frozen peas placed upon your breast. Take Tylenol to reduce pain and fever.

- Have a hot shower and let the water run over your breasts. Apply hot packs to your breasts. Once the hot packs have been applied you can more easily express your excess milk. Only express enough to release the pressure or you will be creating even more milk. Don't worry, engorgement only last a few days and your body will quickly respond to the feeding needs of your baby.
- Cabbage leaves molded into your nursing bra and then frozen can be worn for a short time between feedings for comfort during engorgement.
- When feeding your baby make sure your baby always completely empties the first breast before you go on to the next one. This way you can eliminate any blockages in your breast before they build up. Completely draining the first breast will also increase your milk supply and will increase the weight of your baby at a faster rate.
- Use cold packs on your breasts sparingly as they will reduce your milk supply. You are better off to apply heat and express any extra milk to obtain relief. Pump off only to the point of comfort or else you will increase your milk supply and you will find your breasts filling up again within a half hour.
- If you find any hard lumps the size of a pea in your breast at any time after you have completed a feeding, press down hard on the lump with your thumb or finger and gently work the lump towards your nipple. Make sure your baby sucks that breast completely dry at the next feeding.

- You may find yourself waking up in the middle of the night completely soaked. Keep a supply of clean towels folded by your bed and use one underneath you as you sleep. It is much easier to wash a towel than to change and wash the sheets. Soon your milk will be established and the leaking will stop.

Expressing Your Breast Milk

The best time to express your milk is in the middle of the night or first thing in the morning, before the first feeding. Creating a milk bank can give you peace of mind and the knowledge that you will always have an abundance of milk on hand for your baby. When expressing your milk only one-third of the available milk supply is expressed, only your baby is able to remove the remainder of your milk. When you express your milk that you are naturally increasing the supply available to your baby as supply increases naturally upon demand throughout your breastfeeding relationship.

To defrost frozen breastmilk place the plastic bag into a glass of warm or hot water. It should unthaw within a few minutes. A microwave should never be used to defrost breastmilk.

British Columbia's Children's Hospital has a Breast Milk Service. If you find that you have a great abundance of breast milk, as many women do, you may wish to donate breast milk for premature or ill babies. After you have been screened, the hospital will pick up the breastmilk from your home then the milk is pooled, pasteurized and bacteriologically tested and frozen. This is a labor of love for all involved in Canada and has saved the lives of many babies.

Begin by gently massaging your breast for one minute. Visualize your baby feeding to trigger your mind to bring down your milk. Cup your breast with your fingers on the bottom and your thumb on the top of your breast close to the edge of your areola, which is the brown colored part of your breast. Always keep your thumb in the same position and gently press down and out toward the nipple. Once you find the best spot to release your milk keep your thumb in exactly that spot every time you express your milk. Use the same milking rhythm your baby uses by pressing down and out in short intervals.

You can use a Playtex with plastic liner for breast milk freezing and temporary storage in your refrigerator. When expressing your milk you can use any clean container you happen to have by you.

The first time you express your milk you may express only one ounce or drops. Continue to add to this amount throughout the day and freeze what you have collected at the end each day. Do not add warm milk to frozen milk. Each time you express your milk it will become easier and faster and as you progress in your breastfeeding you will collect more milk each time. To defrost frozen breastmilk place the plastic bag into a glass of warm or hot water. It should unthaw within a few minutes. A microwave should never be used to defrost breastmilk.

Handle your breasts gently at all times especially when you are fully engorged. Your breasts bruise easily. It is not force that brings your milk down but a gentle milking action that will allow you to gently remove excess milk.

Nipple Care

- Always express the last few drops of milk and allow them to air dry naturally on your nipples. Your milk contains natural healing substances that will condition your nipple.
- Never allow your baby to suck on your nipple. For a correct latch your baby must have your nipple and your areola all the way into its mouth.
- Breastfeeding should never hurt. If you are feeling any pain, talk to a female breastfeeding specialist right away.
- Never allow your breasts to become chapped by rubbing against wet fabric or breast pads. Keep an extra pair of cotton breastpads in your purse so that you can quickly change them should they become wet. Washable, cotton breastpads allow air to more easily circulate around your nipples.
- Use A & D Creme, vitamin A and vitamin D in a lanolin creme base, if your nipples become cracked or sore. This cream can also be used on your episiotomy site, your baby's rash, or to heal eczema on your baby's face or body. You can buy this ointment at any large drug store without prescription.
- Your nipples will lose much of their sensitivity after the first month and this sensitivity will come back once you have finished breastfeeding.
- Remain braless as much as possible when at home to keep your nipples dry and to help with the circulation in your breasts.
- Use a hair dryer on a warm setting if your nipples are badly chapped.
- Apply a warm compress for five minutes after a feeding then keep nipples continually dry between feedings.
- Vitamin E oil can also be applied to heal cracked nipples.
- Never use hand or body lotion as they contain ingredients that can harm your baby or give them a distaste and put them off feedings.
- Breastfeed on the side with the least pain to start as your baby will suck more vigorously on that side first. As your baby sucks your nipple will feel better once the milk begins to flow. Your breast milk contains natural healing substances that will work to heal your nipples as your baby feeds.
- If dry or chapped nipples are a continual problem go to a breastfeeding clinic or neighbourhood La Leche League meeting near you to make sure you are properly latching on your baby and that the positioning is correct for your baby.

Thrush

In *Smart Medicine for a Healthier Child: A Practical Reference to Natural and Conventional Treatment for Infants and Children,* you will find a guide to conventional, homeopathic, herbal, nutritional, prevention and acupressure therapy for many disorders. Thrush shows up as white patches inside your baby's mouth, making it difficult for your baby to feed. General information about this condition includes information on related conditions like canker sores, warts, diaper rash, yeast infections and diabetes, which sometimes predisposes to thrush and yeast infections, and nutritional deficiencies that contribute to a general susceptibility to viral, bacterial, or fungal infections in general and of the skin specifically, as well as foods not to eat in case of a yeast infection.

Eating foods rich in vitamin A (carrots), B complex (whole grains, eggs, green beans), vitamin C (tomatoes, greens) folic acid (greens), and eating a whole grain, lean meat, legume, and non-sweet vegetable diet which is inhibitory to yeast can help as well. Refined sugar, flour, and cereal products as well as sweet vegetables and fats, foods which yeast thrives on, should be omitted. Diluted apple cider vinegar with water can also be included for both the baby and mother. Licorice root and ginger tea are also part of the recommended herbal treatment. Contact a breastfeeding consultant for treatment for you and your baby should thrush appear.

Increasing Your Milk Supply

Every mother worries at some time if she has enough milk. Real signs of milk scarcity include a dry diaper two or three hours after feeding or not producing at least eight really wet diapers in a twenty-four hour period. Talk over your concerns with a breastfeeding professional if this should happen.

- Keep in mind that your baby may be crying for reasons other than food. Read the newborn section on crying in this guidebook to find out what your baby's unique sensitivities are and work to temporarily reduce either light, sound or movement in your baby's environment. And you can help your baby to practice self-calming techniques such as sucking on hands, fingers and wrist, focusing and favorite body positioning instead of continual feeding for calming. Training your baby to use other methods to self-calm rather than using your breast to calm will release both of you from becoming completely dependent on each other.
- The easiest way to increase your milk supply is to breastfeed more frequently.
- Give both breasts at each feeding. Make sure each breast is drained before starting on the next one. If your baby still seems hungry, put your baby back onto the first breast to help her get every last drop.

- Do not rigidly limit your baby's sucking time. The composition of milk changes as she sucks the thirst quenching foremilk, like skim milk, and then the more concentrated hindmilk, which is like cream. This hindmilk is very satisfying for your baby and can only be accessed by her when the breast is completely drained to the end.
- Don't offer a bottle instead of the breast. Even if she sucked so recently that you are sure there cannot be any more milk for her there will always be a little left and preventing her from taking it will make your breasts fill up more slowly.
- Don't offer a bottle along with the breast. Frequent breastfeeding will sustain her and cue your breasts to make more milk.
- Breastfeed as often as your baby likes. It doesn't matter if she has to suck very often to keep satisfied, with each feeding your supply is automatically increased. And as your baby grows you will automatically begin to produce greater amounts of breast milk.
- Bringing your baby to bed with you during the night and breastfeeding two or three times during the night will increase your supply. The milk you produce during the night while resting is also very rich and satisfying for your baby.
- Take a walk out in the fresh air before breastfeeding to relax.
- Some mothers have had great success with drinking small amounts of stout beer to restimulate supply.
- If you must leave your baby, express before you leave and while you are away if necessary. The best bet is to find a way to bring your baby with you when you go. You will be surprised at how many people love to see a newborn and your baby will enjoy the outing as well. Breastfed newborns are easily comforted with a feeding and often sleep quite soon after content in your arms.
- If you find that due to personal stress or inadequate nutrition that you do not have the volume of milk you would like, you can purchase the Sunrider "Herb Drink Powder" and mix it up in your blender with fruit and water or milk. This excellent nutritional product can almost double your milk supply within a twenty-four hour period. Then make sure you are eating properly, small meals of nutritional food, throughout the day.
- Keep your fluid intake up throughout the day and evening. The best way to do this is to get a drink for yourself and sip on it every time you breastfeed.
- Rest is also important. Working a short nap into your day will give you the extra energy you need at this time.
- Herb teas that will help to increase your milk supply include blessed thistle, brewer's yeast, red raspberry leaf, marshmallow, or alfalfa for rich milk and added strength for mom.
- Make sure you are taking a mineral supplement. Your baby requires

calcium most of all for the first few years. The calcium will continue to be drawn out of your body's stores and this can cause exhaustion in the mother. Taking good care of yourself during breastfeeding is well worth the end result of a happy mother and baby.

Breastfeeding And Work

You do not have to quit breastfeeding because you are returning to work. It is possible to maintain your milk by breastfeeding your baby in the morning, late afternoon, the evening and night and on the weekends. Supplement with your personal milk bank for the day feedings or try to return home at lunch. Rent a portable breast pump and bring it to work. After you return to your career you will appreciate continuing breastfeeding for the rewards it gives to both of you.

Breastfeeding causes the hormone prolactin to be released in your body, helping you and your baby to reconnect and attach at the end of the day. This hormone will also naturally relax and calm you. Your baby will receive these same benefits and more. Continuing your breastfeeding past your baby's first year will also boost your baby's immune system reducing or eliminating colds, flu and fevers.

New Discoveries on Breastmilk

Excerpted, from, Fit Pregnancy Magazine, *Summer 1995, "Mother's Milk: What's in it for Baby?" written by Janis Graham author of*Breastfeeding Secrets & Solutions, *1993.*

Human breast milk has a full and balanced complement of minerals and vitamins, including calcium, phosphorus, zinc and vitamins B6, B12, C and D. Breast milk also contains a multitude of other components that help the baby grow and thrive. Some of them do double and triple duty. Here's a partial list:

Secretory IgA – This is human milk's most predominant antibody (Ig is short for immunoglobulin). At birth, babies cannot produce their own immunoglobulins. Instead they're protected by transplacental IgC that was transmitted in utero by Mom. But this lasts only a short time. Meanwhile, babies slowly develop the ability to make their own immunoglobulins. At 3 months, babies have a total antibody protection (transplacental IgC plus baby's own antibodies) that's only about 35 percent of what they had at birth. Breast milk's abundant supply of IgA helps fill the gap until babies can take over the entire job of protecting themselves. IgA acts like an intestinal "paint", coating the lining of the baby's gut and binding bacteria and viruses so they can't multiply. After a few hours, this IgA coating is sloughed off, digested as protein and excreted. Each time a baby nurses, he gets a new protective paint job. IgA is believed to play a key role in preventing diarrhea. In addition, whenever a mother is exposed to a bacteria or virus, her body manufactures a specific secretory IgA to protect her. If she's been exposed to a bug, in all likelihood so has her baby, but luckily, her environmentally specific IgA is secreted in her milk and transferred to the baby, bestowing a highly personalized protection.

Lysozyme – This enzyme acts like a powerful little Pac Man in the baby's digestive system. It chops up bacterial cell walls, powerfully and selectively gobbling up disease-carrying bacteria.

Prolactin – Until recently, scientists thought this hormone simply served to regulate Mom's milk production. Its presence in milk was considered a nonfunctional by-product. Research now supports the idea that prolactin helps activate and enhance the infant's immune system. A recent study published in Pediatrics hypothesized that the presence of prolactin and immunoregulatory substances in human milk (and their absence in formula) may be why breastfed babies have a lower risk of ear infection than formula-fed babies.

Sialated Mucins – These combinations of carbohydrate and protein with sialic acid help prevent viral diarrhea-which causes more than 200 infant deaths annually in the United States. Recent research has shown that these mucins can pick up harmful viruses as they pass through the baby's intestine, then transport them out via the feces.

Sialic Acid (also known as n-acetylneuramic acid or NANA). Besides enhancing the protective effect of mucins, NANA is important for normal cell membrane function and brain development. Breast milk contains about 5 to 10 times more sialic acid than formula does.

Complex Oligosaccharides – The blend of these carbohydrates in breast milk is unique. In addition to providing calories, these compounds prevent bacteria from binding to cell surfaces. Several studies have linked oligosaccharides to protection against urinary tract infections.

Lactoferrin – This protein delivers iron directly to where it's needed in the intestinal lining and sequesters unnecessary iron – an important function since many "bad" bacteria can't thrive without extra iron.

Long-Chain Polyunsaturated Fatty Acids – These fatty acids become part of the cell membranes of the infant's nervous system and are thus important to the continued development of the retina and brain. "Striking data indicates that these fatty acids are responsible for the enhanced visual acuity that has been shown to occur in preterm infants who received human milk compared to those who received formula, "notes Judy Hopkinson, PhD., research assistant professor at the USDA Children's Nutrition Research Center at Baylor College of Medicine in Houston.

Bifidobacterium – These "healthy" bacteria, which are capable of destroying parasites, aren't actually present in mother's milk. Instead, certain carbohydrates present only in human milk encourage these bacteria to flourish in the baby's intestinal tract. The benefits of bifidobacterium were highlighted in a recent study conducted at the Johns Hopkins University School of Medicine: When hospitalized babies were given formula with added bifidobacterium, they has a substantially reduced incidence of acute diarrhea disease.

Epidermal Growth Factor – This hormone – like substance is important to the growth and maturation of the linings of the baby's liver, heart, intestines, kidney, pancreas and stomach.

13

Care of the Mother

- Complete rest during the first few weeks will allow your body to recover quickly and naturally.
- Make a new message for your telephone announcing a new boy or girl, the name of your new baby, and the date and time of birth. Let callers know that you both are resting and you will call back when you can.
- Put a note on the door saying that mom and baby are sleeping and to please call to set up a time to visit.
- Find another new mother for support. Another new mom can help you keep your sense of humor as you begin to adjust to your new roles.
- A calm and quiet environment for both mother and baby for the first thirty days is a custom respected in many tribal societies.
- Take a quick shower or bath every day during the first two weeks. Bring your baby into the bathroom, after a feeding, and lay her down on the bathroom mat if it makes you feel more secure. Your baby will enjoy the noise and steam from the bath and you will appreciate the time to care for yourself.
- Get plenty of rest during the first thirty days. You deserve it. It is easy to feel overwhelmed if you are tired from not getting enough sleep.
- If you feel that you are bleeding excessively, one pad per hour or more, call your doctor immediately.
- If you find a foul odor coming from you, call your doctor immediately.
- In the first few days you may pass larger blood clots. This is normal.
- For hemorrhoids try Vaseline on the affected area between medication applications to avoid irritation.
- You should find your bleeding beginning to taper off and change from bright red, to brown to a light clear discharge after a few weeks. Bed rest is extremely important to help your body to heal itself. If you find yourself with a bright red discharge all of a sudden, slow down your activities, and bring your baby back to bed with you for two or three days.

- Each time you urinate or change your pad use this opportunity to use a warm water rinse on your vaginal area. A sports drink bottle with a flip-top can be used to spray warm water as you sit on the toilet. Keep your vaginal area as clean as possible for the first two weeks. Adding Calendula tincture to the warm water rinse can help soothe and heal.
- A light application of Vaseline can also help to soothe an episiotomy area and ease pain upon urination. Clean this away thoroughly afterwards with a warm water rinse.
- Aloe vera gel can help with itching from an episiotomy site.
- Calendula tincture on pads stored in the freezer can give quick relief from itching at an episiotomy site.
- Arrange to have a sitz bath or Epsom salt bath if episiotomy stitches are bothering you.
- Use A & D Creme, found at drugstores, to lightly coat cuts or tears in your vaginal area to avoid pain upon urination and to help healing.
- Sleep at every opportunity you find.
- Rest and eat well.
- Set up a half hour or an hour once a day all for yourself. Soak in the tub, read a good book, write a letter to a friend or take the time to balance your checkbook. If your partner is unable to watch your baby for this time, find an older neighbor or hire a young girl for an hour out of each day. It will be just what you need to recharge and appreciate your baby after a break.
- Relax and remember that your baby is new at this too – you are learning together.
- Don't be afraid to ask for help and also to let people know when you've had enough help.
- Ask your caregiver to give most of the baby care over to you, have your caregiver focus on the many others things that need to be done, especially running errands and cooking. Being a parent takes practice, doing the same things over and over and by the second week you will feel much more competent and natural with your new work when you've had this time with your baby.
- You do not have to be overly strong during your home recovery. Ask your doctor for pain relief if necessary.
- If you find cramping a problem as your womb returns to its former size drink raspberry leaf tea, purchased at any health food store, to recondition your uterus. Daily light massage to your lower stomach area can also help to reduce cramping and help to shrink your uterus. Catnip tea can also help with afterpains.
- If you have not had a bowel movement in three days you might want to

try an enema. An enema will soften your bowel movement so that you are less likely to disturb any surgery site, if you have one.

- Contact a school for massage if you are feeling pain in your neck or shoulders. Many schools allow the students to practice on you at a much reduced price and you can bring your baby along with you. Feed your baby before your appointment and bring your baby into the massage school in your car seat and you will easily have an hour or two of uninterrupted time just for you.

- If you have trouble urinating let your doctor know immediately.

- Make a plan to care for yourself immediately after the first morning feeding for your baby. Your baby will usually be contented and sleepy after the first feeding and you may find this is the only time for personal grooming during the day. Have a shower or bath, put on your make-up if you usually wear it and spend extra time on your hair. When you care for yourself first you will find that you have more to give to your baby.

- Watch out for the "super woman" syndrome. Yes, the cleaning can wait. Take the extra moments in the day to relax, recharge and get to know your new baby. Use shortcuts whenever you can. Leave the laundry in the basket when necessary. Put your feet up whenever you can and have short power naps. Your body has amazing recuperative abilities and allowing yourself to rest frequently will give your body what it needs at this time.

- If you feel overwhelmed with the dependency of your new baby talk to someone who can understand what you are feeling. This may be your husband, your mother, your best friend or your doctor or midwife. These feelings are natural. You are dealing with new routines, exhaustion and hormones. It is important to reassure yourself that most people will feel overwhelmed by a new baby. Knowing that you are not alone and having a support network of other new mothers can do wonders for your self-confidence and your self-esteem.

- Join a weekly parents group to add to the friends you already know. Your single friends won't always understand the depth of commitment needed to care for a baby and build a family. Very few people have 24 hour jobs unless they happen to be a parent. Find another new mother to complain to, be empathetic to, and laugh with as you both experience the joys and challenges motherhood.

- Continue to take your prenatal vitamins for the first six months after your baby is born, especially if you are breastfeeding. Your body has given a tremendous amount and uses up many of its nutritional stores throughout your pregnancy. By continuing to take your vitamins you will be giving back to your body and creating reserves for the months ahead.

- Choose one day a week or one day a month to reconnect with who you were before. Use this special time to reconnect with your mate, join a dance club, visit single girlfriends, or any favorite activity you have that doesn't scream mommy. This means no scouting out playschools or shopping for baby clothes. A happy mom equals a happy baby. Taking time to be you again will help you to reestablish your equilibrium.
- Take time for yourself, doing things you used to do even if it's only a few minutes here and there because if Mom falls apart, the whole family seems to.
- Your new life will fall into place if you take one step at a time. Get lots of emotional support, accept any offers to help and delegate "duties" if possible to get the rest you deserve and require.
- Recent research from *Mothering The New Mother*, by Sally Placksin, 1994, is now showing that postpartum adjustment for a first-time mother realistically takes six months to a year. It takes at least a year to build a working family. Fathers experience the same length of adjustment with a new baby. Create a good support network of other new mothers and families to assist you with enjoying this exciting transition. Many new parents are finding the recent proliferation of parenting classes to be worthwhile and supportive for adapting to the new changes.

14

Newborn Care Tips

The First Day

- Keeping your newborn close to you at all times during the first few weeks helps to build a bond of love and trust between you.
- Your baby is experiencing a profound adjustment as she is seeing, feeling and hearing our world for the first time. The best thing you can do for your baby is spend the day together in bed, only an arm's length away. Your baby has gone through a physically tiring labor and delivery. Your body also has gone through a tremendous strain, even more so if you have had any medical interventions with either your labor or delivery and your body is now providing colostrum and creating your breastmilk. Taking the next one or two weeks to rest will help your body to completely heal and for your milk supply to be created. Some cases of postnatal depression are rooted in the first few weeks home due to inadequate rest of the mother. Ask now and take all the assistance that is offered. You deserve to be cared for during this time.
- Not all women experience "love at first sight" especially if they have had a difficult delivery. This is completely normal. Don't feel guilty. Over time you fall madly in love with your precious baby.
- Your newborn is genetically designed to look more like your partner in the first few months of life. Most mothers are surprised at the great likeness in their babies to their partners and have trouble finding any likeness at all to themselves. Your baby will change to look more like you after the first month or two. This process is nature's way to assist both partners in continuing to bond to the new member of the family.
- Keep the lights in your home dim for the first day and noise to a minimum. Entertain any guests in your bedroom and ask all guests to keep their voices low. Don't feel you have to let anyone other than your partner handle or hold your baby. Explain that just for today, you are

keeping the house as quiet as possible.

- Breastfeed as often as you have the opportunity in your baby's first hours. Your baby will be awake for three hours or more directly after birth and will be the most alert for the longest time in the days to come. Some newborns will sleep for twelve to twenty-four hours after their first alert period.

- If you have any breastfeeding difficulties on the first day immediately contact your nurse, midwife, lactation consultant or breastfeeding mom to voice your concerns. Many breastfeeding challenges can be solved on the telephone. The most challenging problems are an improper latch or the position of the baby at the breast. Taking care of small problems before they become big problems will help you to easily become a great breastfeeding team.

- No matter how many pacifiers or soothers you are given for gifts do not use them. Studies are showing a direct link to pacifiers and ear infections in infants. A pacifier will cause your baby to be unable to communicate her needs to you and your baby will not be able to access it for herself when she needs soothing. Babies have also been shown to self-wean early when they are given pacifiers. If you are tempted to use one to forestall crying, see the crying and colic section of this guide for alternate methods for soothing a crying baby. Pacifiers also cause more difficulty with efficient feeding as your baby's jaw can become quite sore from the continual, instinctual sucking action caused by pacifiers. Babies who are given free and easy access to their hands in the first year rarely suck on their fingers or thumbs past the first year.

- Keep your baby's hands free from clothing and blankets at all times. Roll up the sleeves on jumpers and place the blanket only up to your baby's waist, leaving hands and arms completely free and available to your baby. If you are swaddling your baby keep those hands and arms free, wrapping the blanket under your baby's arms. From the first day, encourage your baby to suck on her fist, arm or fingers, just as your baby did in your womb. Fists, fingers and thumbs are available, clean and your baby will always be able to find them for comfort and security.

- Try a nail file for your baby's fingernails instead of clippers. Clippers are difficult to manage with a newborn and you run the risk of cutting the skin. You may need to file the nails on a daily basis as they will grow rapidly. Think of your baby's fingers and thumbs as your baby's best tools and keep them in good condition and available at all times.

- Give others the opportunity to hold your baby. Watch carefully how they hold, soothe and talk to your baby. You will get new ideas on how to be with your baby.

- Help your partner to change, hold and comfort your baby from the first day. Learn together what works best for your baby and share with each other your new discoveries of what works best.
- Set aside two days for friends and relatives to see your new baby. Having everyone over at once is easier for you and your baby.
- When placing your baby on the sofa, place your baby's back or side against the back of your sofa so that your baby feels more secure and less overwhelmed with such a large space around her. This also works well in the crib or cradle.
- Purchase a foam holder to assist your baby in sleeping on the side instead of on her back or stomach. You can also use a rolled towel or receiving blanket. This has been found to be the safest position for your baby while sleeping. Should your baby vomit or spit up while sleeping, there would be less risk of choking.
- Keep all toys, pillows, down quilts, stuffed animals and the like out of your baby's crib or bassinet until your baby is at least one year of age to insure that fresh air easily circulates around your baby at all times.
- Babies can be overstimulated by anxious parents trying to rock, burp, soothe a newborn who just wants to be left alone. If your baby is fed, burped, dry, and warm, give your baby at least two minutes to vent and remove outside stimulus as in dimming the lighting, turning down the television or radio, and slowing down or stopping movement. You will find that your newborn craves a quiet environment when she is overtired. Peace and quiet is one of the greatest sources of comfort you can give your newborn in the first few months.

Sleeping

Consider having your baby sleep beside you. Mothers have been sleeping in the same bed as their infants for centuries. Sharing your bed with your baby has many benefits:

- Your baby learns sleep and breathing patterns by being near you throughout the night. The carbon dioxide you breath out also helps your baby to breath better and stimulates breathing as well.
- Breastfeeding in the middle of the night is much easier if your baby is in bed with you as it won't disrupt your sleeping patterns.
- It is less upsetting for your baby to sleep with you initially as your baby will not have to cry loud, or a long time to get your attention.
- Premature babies or other babies who were separated from their mothers at the hospital may attach more easily when they sleep with their mothers. This type of close contact will help your baby thrive.
- Safety first. Never sleep with your baby if you are drinking alcohol or

taking drugs. Never let your baby sleep on a waterbed. Never place your baby on a bed that has a loose headboard or sideboards.

- If you feel uncomfortable, or if you, your baby or your partner are not sleeping well in this arrangement, set things up to suit yourself. You may want to use a cradle or bassinet next to your bed or to place the crib in your bedroom. A crib or cradle in your room beside the bed gives both of you the benefits from sleeping together for the first few months.

- Decide on your own time when to move your baby out of your bed. Have a small wicker basket or cradle at your bedside and gradually have your baby sleep there for part of the night. Make changes gradually so that everyone adjusts easily.

- Purchase a foam holder to assist your baby in sleeping on the side or back instead of on her stomach. You can also use a rolled towel or receiving blanket. This has been found to be the safest position for your baby while sleeping. Should your baby vomit or spit up while sleeping, there would be less risk of choking.

- Keep all toys, pillows, stuffed animals and the like out of your baby's crib or bassinet until your baby is at least one year of age to insure that fresh air easily circulates around your baby.

- With more babies sleeping on their backs now, you may want to place your baby on her tummy at playtime to help round out your baby's head.

Bottle-Feeding

- Cow's milk is ideal for calves but it is not the natural food for babies. It contains too little sugar and the wrong kind of fat. Its protein makes indigestible solid curds in the baby's stomach. Babies under one year should not be fed on any kind of unmodified cow's milk. Babies need a breastmilk substitute for the entire first year if they are not breastfed.

- If you are not breastfeeding you must give your baby additional mineral supplements with an infant formula. In Canada and the United States our dogs are fed a formula with 40 added minerals. Laboratory rats and mice are fed a formula with 28 added minerals. Every infant formula on the market sold in the 1990s has fewer than 12 added minerals. Extra mineral support is critical for the health of your baby. Liquid colloidal minerals added to your baby's formula will give your baby the over 60 added minerals that humans need for proper physical development.

- Don't be mislead by the advertising of the multi-million dollar baby formula companies. Issues such as price gouging, unfair advertising practices, monopolization of the market, and inferior formulation have only recently come to light. You can lobby to have the makers of infant formula upgrade their product by calling the toll-free number listed on the packaging.

- A new baby, especially one who is not breastfed, has few defenses against common germs. Formula, especially formula which is room temperature is an ideal breeding ground for germs. So while she will pick up a few off her own fingers and deal with them perfectly well, she will pick up an overwhelming number from a bottle which has been left standing around in a warm room. Gastroenteritis is still one of the most common reasons for babies being admitted to the hospital. Keep your baby's formula as free from bacteria as possible.

- To keep your formula free from bacteria, wash your hands before handling the formula or equipment. Use a sterile formula and keep the can tightly covered and refrigerated once it has been opened. Sterilize everything you use in measuring, mixing or storing the made-up formula. Sterilize bottles, nipples and nipple covers. Keep the formula cold until your baby wants it. Never put warm formula in a thermos or electric bottle warmer. Throw away any formula your baby leaves behind. Don't try to save that half bottle for next time and don't pour the now unsterile remains back into your jar of sterilized formula in the refrigerator.

- If you do not have access to sterilizing equipment, cup feed or dropper feed your baby instead of using a bottle.

- When you combine formula powder or liquid concentrate with boiled water you are constructing food and most of your baby's drink. If you do it in exactly the proportions the manufacturer suggests, your baby will get the right amount of food and the right amount of water. Always follow the manufacturer's instructions exactly.

- You cannot make it better by putting in just a little extra powder or more thirst quenching by adding extra water. If you add too much powder, the formula will be too strong. Your baby will get too much protein, too much fat, too much salt, and not enough water. She will get fat because you are giving her too many calories and thirsty because you are giving her too much salt. Because she is thirsty, she will cry, and because she cries you will give her another bottle. If that bottle is too strong, she will be even more thirsty. The result can be a baby who cries a lot, does not seem terribly well or happy, puts on a lot of weight, and seems to need a lot of feeding.

- Never carry warm formula. It is a dangerously ideal breeding ground for bacteria. Carry the baby's formula icy cold from the refrigerator. Keep it that way by putting the sterile sealed bottles in an insulated bag or by burying them in ice cubes in a plastic bag. Warm the bottles as you need them by standing them in hot water from a thermos for a few minutes. If you are going to need more bottles than you can safely keep cold, measure formula powder into empty sterile bottles and seal. Mix with boiled water from a thermos as you need each one. Always carry at least one more feeding than you think you will need during the trip.

- How often do you feed a bottle-fed baby? Formula should be offered whenever the baby seems to be hungry and the feeding should only be stopped when eager sucking ceases. Don't try to push her to take more than she really wants. Your newborn's stomach is the size of her closed hand and will require small meals quite frequently for the first few months. Each baby has their own individual feeding requirements.

- A newborn is used to having her food needs continually replenished by transfusion feeding in the womb. While your baby gets used to this new method of feeding she may be hungry at irregular and frequent intervals. If you offer her a bottle whenever she seems hungry, she will only take the amount she needs. If she drinks it all you can assume she needed it. If she takes a little, the comfort of sucking and of your care will make her feel better. If she drinks none, what have you lost? If you meet these irregular demands willingly, they will stop by themselves in a few weeks. Do not put a newborn on any feeding schedule for this reason. After a few months your baby's unique feeding pattern will evolve on its own. So don't fall into the trap of thinking that if you feed your baby whenever she seems hungry she will get into the habit of demanding food frequently.

- Being physically close to you during feedings is just as important to the bottle-fed baby as to the breastfed baby. Always give her the bottle while she is cradled in your arms. Eating is a social occasion for us all including your baby. Choose a chair that supports your back and arms while your feet are flat on the floor. Always bottle-feed your baby with her head higher than her body in an upright or semi-upright position. Do not let your baby bottle-feed lying down as the fluids can accumulate in the ear canal causing ear infections. If you are bottle-feeding in your bed, place your arm under your baby's head to raise it up.

- When your baby stops sucking or when the feeding is finished you may want to burp your baby. Hold her upright against your shoulder, rub her back or pat it gently. If she has not burped after three minutes, she does not need to.

- If you find your baby either gaining too much weight or not gaining enough weight on your dairy-based formula you may want to switch to a soy-based baby formula for a thirty-day period. Many babies are milk intolerant and have difficulties digesting and eliminating the protein from a dairy-based formula. Read the section in this guide that deals with allergies and food intolerances if this is the case.

Diapering

- Make a game out of changing your baby's diaper and clothes. Smile at your baby. Laugh when your baby makes a big poop. Make this a fun time for your baby by taking an extra few minutes to talk to your baby, ask your baby questions and listen for responses, give a short massage on legs or arms, or to comment on your plans for the day. Your baby will cherish these times together with you and will also enjoy your undivided attention.

- Place an oversized mirror on the wall beside your baby's change table. Your baby will enjoy the reflection of both of you from the first day and will be fascinated at the changing images.

- Changing your baby in the bathroom will give you a mirror and water facilities.

- Keep a spray bottle of water at your change table. Spray your baby's bottom with water after bowel movements and your baby will clean up easily. Use the corners of the last diaper to clean off. Use as many diaper wipes as necessary to be sure diaper area is completely clean, as anything left on the skin will cause a rash. Give another quick spray after using the diaper wipes to get every last trace of soap off.

- If you are not using diaper wipes, a quick rinse in the sink can clean your baby's bottom in a minute.

- Don't change your baby when your baby is hungry.

- Expect your baby's first bowel movements to be black and tar-like, the next movements will be green, and then onto a seedy, mustard yellow. You may wish to use disposable diapers for the first two weeks of large bowel movements. Try buying the next size larger than newborn for complete coverage of these messy bowel movements.

- When possible, let your baby's bottom air dry by leaving the diaper and other clothes off for a short time by placing your baby on a disposable waterproof pad.

- If your diapers leak, change your diapers to a bigger size or to another brand.

- Breastfed babies sometimes go for a few days between bowel movements. As long as the bowel movement is still mustard yellow and has a soft texture, everything is fine.

- If your baby's skin is very sensitive try using natural aloe vera gel instead of powders or sticky creams. Make sure the gel is completely dry before putting diaper on to be assured that the protection will stay on the skin and not rub off on the diaper. You can also use this gel for prickly heat rashes.

- A & D Creme, found in any drugstore without prescription, works extremely well on diaper rash. This ointment is natural, inexpensive and offers great value for your money.

- If your diaper cream is not working as you would like, switch brands until you find one you like. When you find one that works, purchase the largest size to save money. It is not necessary to use diaper cream all the time.
- Try natural Corn Starch, found in the grocery store, for a natural baby powder that helps prevent diaper rashes. Keep all powders away from your baby's reach so that they are not accidently breathed into your or your baby's lungs.
- Your baby should not continually have rashes. Check your diaper wipes or diapers to see if they are causing any sensitivity to your baby's skin. Look at the foods your baby is consuming: sometimes a rash is brought on by food reactions to dairy, fruits, bananas, etc. Remove or replace that food with another and see if the condition clears up. Disposable diapers can also cause a sensitivity. If you are using cloth diapers try using a detergent purchased as a health food grocery store that has no dyes, phosphates, or chemicals. Make sure you presoak your diapers in dissolved Borax to change the acidic environment to alkaline.
- Alternative cotton disposable diapers from Tushies are a great alternative to plastic, chemical-filled diapers. To order in Canada call 1-888-270-2027.
- For a diaper rash that just won't go away try "Bactroban" 2% antibiotic ointment. It is available without a prescription. Use three times a day for two days. If it will work for your baby, you will notice a marked improvement in two days. Use sparingly, for a maximum of three days at a time. If a rash just won't go away take your baby in to see your doctor.

Crying & Colic – How to Help Your Baby to Stop Crying

All crying in the first year should be attended to immediately.

Crying is your baby's only method of communication with you.

If your newborn is crying constantly throughout the day and night, take your baby to the hospital or to your doctor immediately for a thorough checkup to assure yourself that your baby is well.

Some newborns are more sensitive to their environment than others. Should this be the case for your baby, the following suggestions may be of great assistance in creating a calm and soothing environment for you and your baby.

Thousands of parents have used the following self-calming method for their newborns with great success. Many see results in as early as seven days on the program. Expect your best results to come after you have used the program for thirty days. Never shake a crying baby as this can permanently damage the brain of your baby and will not stop the crying anyway.

If your newborn has a pattern of crying non-stop for three or four hours, usually in the evening, wearing the both of you down, you may want to try the following to help your baby to stop crying. A newborn's world is loud, bright and similar to a nonstop ride at the carnival. Amazing new discoveries in the field of newborn care are now showing us that most crying in newborns is due to over-stimulation.

1. If, after your baby is fed, changed and warm, your baby is still crying, try taking your baby immediately into a quiet, dimly lit room. Turn down the lights, turn down the noise, and slow down your movement and activity.
2. Hold your baby's face and body away from you, facing your baby outward so that your baby can visually focus on something in the room.
3. Free your baby's hands and wrists from clothing and bring both of your baby's hands gently up towards your baby's face so that your baby can either focus on or suck on fingers, thumbs or wrist.
4. During this process it is best for the adult to remain silent.
5. As your baby begins to calm look for reasons for the crying. For example when has your newborn had the last opportunity to rest undisturbed or what activities came before the crying.
6. While you are in the quiet, darkened room either hold your baby or place your baby in her favorite body position on your bed with a hand gently massaging either back or bottom of the feet. Look for signs of your baby beginning to calm on her own. Always make sure that your baby has easy access to her hands and wrists by rolling up the sleeves to the elbow and swaddling under the arms leaving the hands free.

As you get to know your baby, look to see what disturbs your baby the most when your baby is overstimulated. Is the most disturbing factor too much sound, light or movement?

If sound upsets your baby, stop talking, and turn down the volume on your television or stereo. Some babies find movement disruptive when they are overstimulated. If movement affects your baby, lay your baby down beside you and cease movement and activity until your baby begins to calm. If light disturbs your baby the most, immediately dim the lights or go into a darkened room. Using all three of these techniques at once in the beginning will allow you to obtain quick results while you are discovering your baby's unique sensitivities and abilities.

All newborns have instinctual self-calming techniques that help them to deal with the overload of new experiences they have every day. Given the opportunity your baby may instinctively begin to self-calm by doing one or all of the following:

1. Suck on wrist, hand, finger or thumb.
2. Focus visually on a blank space, white wall, or hand and fingers.
3. Have a favorite calming body position like laying on the back, or stomach, side or in a sitting up position.

- When you see that your baby is beginning to self-calm by either sucking, focusing or laying in a particular position, watch your baby without disturbing the process. If your newborn has had an extremely stressful day filled with activities, noise and movement you may see your baby work at self-calming for thirty minutes or more. By standing back and not giving your baby further stimulation at this time you are allowing your baby to create the confidence that comes naturally with a self-calmed baby. It is a great feeling for the parent to know that they are assisting their baby in what is natural for every baby.
- Make sure your baby has at least two quiet periods during the day to nap without noise or distractions. Highly sensitive babies need this quiet time everyday to de-stress.
- The best time to practice self-calming techniques with your baby is in the mornings. Late in the day and early evenings can be trying until your baby learns to rely on these skills. It may take four weeks or so for you and your baby to master these techniques and your patience and guidance will greatly assist your baby in developing this skill at this time. During the first thirty days you will have some setbacks and there may be times when your baby is unable to self-soothe. This is natural and should be expected as both parents and baby develop this skill.
- Using pacifiers, automatic swings, car rides, rocking and walking or whatever else you may have heard of will only delay your baby's ability to develop this skill of self-calming. It is far preferable to take the time now to assist your sensitive baby to be calm and relaxed. Many parents wish they had these skills for themselves. In our fast paced world we all need to acquire the ability to relax and release the stress from our busy days.
- Often your baby will cry today because of the activities that happened the day before. Review where you went and what you did the day before and then reduce your daily activity level with your baby for a week or two while you are helping your baby with self-calming. Have the groceries sent in, delay errands or have someone else pick things up for you, pay your bills by mail and postpone whatever isn't essential during this period of time. This will help you to see what unique combination of sensitivities your baby has and will give you more immediate results with the program.
- As a protective skill your baby is also born with an instinctual ability to play "possum". Many people are amazed to see a baby peacefully sleeping in the midst of a noisy party, such as a christening or baby shower. In this instance your newborn is using an innate ability to shut out all distractions in an attempt to deal with an overload of stimulus. Using this skill is very tiring for a baby as it takes much more energy than

sleeping. You will probably notice that your sensitive baby will be more agitated the next day as a result of the party. Babies will usually lose the skill to play "possum" from the age of six weeks to three months. This skill can be lost in a day when a previously happy and content baby becomes a crying baby. This is the end of the honeymoon period for most babies and parents and an excellent time to encourage your baby to self-calm using this natural, instinctual ability.

- Some mothers stop breastfeeding at six weeks if they have been using extra feedings to calm their newborn. Breastfeeding is a natural way for your baby to use instinctual self-calming methods as it combines sucking, focusing and favorite body position. Unfortunately soon the mother begins to resent continuous and prolonged feedings and the infant soon resents being offered food as the only solution for every problem, just as we would if someone put food into our mouth every time we were frustrated, angry or tired.

- Researchers once felt that at this critical period of time, when your baby is no longer able to play "possum", the baby was going through a growth spurt. After measuring hundreds of babies during this period, and no measurable growth appearing in the babies, we have discovered that the reality is that your baby is actually losing one skill, the ability to play possum and tune everything out, to rely more frequently upon and to develop the other instinctual skills of sucking, focusing and body positioning for self-calming.

- As you get to know your baby's unique sensitivities you may notice that if your baby is overly sensitive to loud noises or talking when overtired, your baby will also probably love music in any form when rested and relaxed. Then communicating with your baby through nursery rhymes and songs, lullabies, sharing your favorite music or buying a musical mobile for your crib, children's tape player and tapes or any musical toy will help you to experience your baby's world from their point of view.

- You can get to know the baby who is sensitive visually by noticing the shadows on the wall as your baby is watching the various light patterns, talking about the light that has caught your baby's eye, pointing out the stars at night or a street light in the evening. Your visually oriented baby may enjoy going to movies, watching you while feeding, sitting up on your lap and being able to see what is going on in the world around them. By catching your baby's attention when your baby is noticing something you will have a short opportunity to explain what it is or what it does. Taking 30 seconds at a time to notice what your baby sees and talking about it will encourage your baby's curiosity and your baby will feel more connected to you.

- A baby who is sensitive to activity may prefer being placed in a favorite sleeping position with a firm hand placed on the back or stomach for a few minutes before sleep. This may calm your baby and will slow down the activity level. Your baby will greatly enjoy being free of encumbrances and holding devices. The best place for this baby is a large blanket on the floor with plenty of encouragement to move about. This baby loves to have you on the floor beside them when playing and will enjoy any kind of physical activity when rested and calm.

- Your baby may have one or any combination of the above sensitivities. You can easily discover for yourself the unique way your baby perceives our world by becoming aware of these traits in your baby. Teach your family and alternate caregivers these self-calming methods and let them know what you've discovered about your baby and they will be as amazed as you will be with the effectiveness of this program.

- As you get to know your baby, you will begin to know how long your baby can cry before your baby is unable to calm. When settling your baby down for a nap your baby will initially protest by crying. Each day you bring your baby in for a nap the time of crying should become shorter. If you feel your baby may be crying for a particular reason or wish to ease your mind, go in and pick up your baby while staying in the room. If your baby immediately stops crying you will know that your baby was able to self-calm and that you may have entered the room too soon. If your baby takes a long time to calm after you have picked your baby up then your baby has a shorter time in which they can cry before they will self-calm. It is a great advantage to a baby to be able to put themselves to sleep without crutches like pacifiers, bottles and frequent visits throughout the evening, and your baby's skill at falling asleep alone will increase with self-calming practice.

- As your baby increases her skill level of self-calming and you learn what your baby's sensitivities are, you will find that it becomes easier to know what your baby needs from you at any particular time. When your baby has been fed within the last two hours, is dry and clean and warm, you will look at your watch to see when the last time your baby had a chance to "de-stress" from daily events by napping. We often forget how noisy, bright, and fast-moving our world is. Everything is new to your baby and giving your baby a chance to slowly adjust to the world can be the best gift you give your newborn.

- A crying baby adds stress to your family relationship. Take the time to carefully watch your baby for signs of self-calming and encourage your baby in each step. Working together as a team will create a calm and loving environment for you both and your baby will learn self-calming techniques that can last a lifetime.

For further study of this amazing new research on why baby's cry you can read *The Self-Calmed Baby*, by William A.H. Sammons, 1989. Every baby should come with crying instructions. This program often yields more than a 90% success rate when field tested with new parents and new babies.

Baby's First Bath

- You can wait to bath your baby until after the umbilical cord has fallen off.
- Wash your baby's hands and face each morning with a warm washcloth and keep your baby's bottom clean with your spray bottle of water or a quick rinse in the sink, keeping this area spotlessly clean especially after a bowel movement.
- When you feel ready you may wish to bring your baby into the big bathtub with you for the first bathing experience. Lean back against the tub with your thighs at a slant. Place your baby on the slant of your legs with only your baby's feet in the water. Talk and smile at your baby to reduce any tension from this new experience. Use a washcloth to bring water up from the tub and over your baby. If you like breastfeed your baby while in the tub to make this a memorable experience for both of you.
- Later, when bathing your baby, you may wish to wash your baby's hair over the sink or small tub while she is still clothed, then continue to undress and bathe the rest of your baby. This can reduce the fear of this new experience and will keep your baby warmer and more comfortable.
- Europeans bathe their babies two or three times a week instead of daily to prevent dry skin. Your baby will not require a daily bath until she starts crawling.

How Install Your Car Seat

Excerpted from Kacz's Kids newsletter, Car Seats – Are Your Babies Safe? *Kacz's Kids is a large retailer of quality infant clothing and baby accessories.*

Most parents believe they are doing all they can to prevent their children from being injured in a car accident. Transport Canada found in their own study that six out of ten children are at risk because of neglect to use or incorrect use of car seats and seat belts. Police, the province and public safety groups have launched a zero tolerance blitz to make certain children are safe. Drivers who fail to make sure the children in their car are secured safely risk incurring tickets for violation of safety laws and they must attend mandatory re-education instruction sessions.

The most common problem with poor car seat safety remains improperly installed tether anchor bolts. A tether bolt is required in all Canadian provinces and is a bolt attached to the rear deck frame, not just the upholstery, of the car. A strap from the car seat is then attached to the bolt. Since 1989 all cars in Canada must have a hole drilled by the manufacturer that accommodates this bolt. To find the bolt, look for the plastic dome that covers it. To install the bolt, just pop out the dome. If you have an earlier model than 1989, then you would have to take your vehicle in to a service center to have the hole drilled.

Deciding which seat to purchase is largely a matter of determining your child's weight: Infant Car Seats are for babies weighing less than 9 kg/20 lbs and should be rear facing with the infant's head protected and supported by the back of their infant seat. It is a Canadian law that your child be securely fastened into their car seat in the correct manner. NEVER PLACE A CAR SEAT OR A CHILD IN THE FRONT SEAT OF A VEHICLE THAT IS EQUIPPED WITH AIRBAGS.

Convertible Forward Facing Seats are for children between 9-18 kg/20-40 lbs. The seat must be properly anchored to the car with a tether strap and bolt plus the car seat belt. The harness straps go over the shoulders and not under the arms. The shoulder straps are secured with a shoulder harness clip supplied by the manufacturer and placed at chest level. Again, this is a Canadian law that your child is secured in this manner.

Sales personnel are trained to offer you the best product available but the most important person for knowledge is yourself. Don't assume you know how a car seat works or any other product that involves a child's safety. Always read your owner's manual for complete and proper instructions.

Establishing A Night-Time Ritual

- Remember even a newborn, one day old, can sleep for six straight hours.
- When your baby awakens during the middle of the night, do not change the diaper unless you absolutely have to.
- Keep all lights dim. Use a night light close to your bed, in the hall and in your baby's room for easier night-time navigation.
- Do not talk to your baby in the middle of the night and your baby will soon realize that night is for sleeping not visiting.
- Tell your baby that it is time to sleep when you lay your baby down.
- If your breasts become completely engorged at night, and your baby has not yet awakened, wake your baby up gently and feed. You are a breastfeeding team and you deserve to be comfortable as well. Or keep a clean glass by your bedside and express just until you feel comfortable.
- Expect at least one middle-of-the-night feeding for the first few months. Keeping your baby in your bedroom will help everyone to get back to sleep faster.
- Many babies will cry out in the middle of the night and then settle themselves down. Wait for two minutes before you attend to your baby to see if your baby goes back to sleep on their own.
- Have your baby in your bed or beside your bed for ease of feeding at night. To avoid turning on the lights, place a finger on your nipple and

bring baby's mouth to your breast, as this will help your baby to latch on in the dark.

- Do not keep your baby awake during the day, hoping this will tire your baby out at night. An over-tired baby has a hard time getting to sleep. Let your baby sleep throughout the day and early evening if needed. It is not necessary to awaken your newborn for feedings during daytime naps as this practice conditions your baby to relate sleeping and eating. Your newborn needs uninterrupted sleeping periods to recharge fully and will awaken naturally when ready.
- Sleep during the daytime, preferably at least two naps, a nap in the morning and in the afternoon of a few hours duration in a quiet room or in your arms, is the best answer for most newborns. Make your baby's nap the most important time of the day and work to schedule other events around this time. This way your newborn will receive the periods of quiet and calmness a very new baby needs, and you will get a much needed break to recharge your batteries as well.
- Sometimes babies awaken during the night because their feet are cold even though the rest of them is warm. Putting a pair of socks on under a sleeper or nightgown can help to keep your baby at the right temperature all night long.
- Establishing a night-time ritual can also consist of a warm bath, feeding or rocking, playing a wind-up mobile or music box, reading a story or anything you choose to do consistently before bed.

Jaundice

For mild jaundice, breastfeed your baby as much as possible in the first three days to eliminate or prevent jaundice. The colostrum that is created before the breast milk is designed to help your baby to expel the first black, green and then yellow stools. Do not feed your baby water as a remedy for jaundice. Place your baby on the carpet in front of a sunny window with only a diaper on for ten or fifteen minutes a day, shading your baby's eyes from direct sunlight, or place your crib or cradle in a sunny spot in the room. Consult your health team if your baby has lethargy, is refusing to feed, or any other symptoms associated with jaundice.

Cradle Cap

- For flakes, massage a little mineral oil into hair and shampoo out. If your baby has a tougher case, where you can see patches of yellow or brown scales in the scalp, purchase a high quality Primrose Oil, from your health food store. Puncture the gel caps and massage into your baby's scalp every day for one week.

- Olive oil, castor oil, or calendula cream can also be used topically to remove the scales. Apply directly onto your baby's scalp, massage in and let soak for 15 minutes. Apply firm but gentle pressure with a fine toothed comb, loosen and comb out the scales and then shampoo.
- Some mothers are finding that reducing their own sugar intake when breastfeeding can help tremendously in reducing or eliminating cradle cap.
- Some doctors recommend a weak solution of cortisone cream for extreme cradle cap that spreads in small patches to the body. Cortisone will thin the skin if used extensively. Instead try Vitamin A and D creme on any patches that may occur on your baby's body or calendula cream which can be purchased in a health food store.
- Comb your baby's hair every day even if your baby has only fine down. This will help with scalp circulation.

Umbilical Cord Care

Soak a Q-tip in rubbing alcohol, lightly pull up cord, and run the Q-tip around the interior of the belly button making sure to get all the way around. Do this every time you change your baby's diaper. If the cord starts to smell, or if you can see that it is getting infected, see your doctor right away.

Talking to Your Baby

Studies show that talking to your baby from the first day can help to create a more alert baby. Ask your baby questions and wait for a response. Say, "Did you have a good sleep?" Then wait 30 seconds for a response. Then come up with your own answer for your baby.

- Use your baby's proper name whenever possible in your sentences.
- Copy out loud the various grunts, squeaks and sounds of your baby. Your partner will be excellent at this. Soon you will have a language together all your very own. Whether you speak your baby's language of grunts and squeaks or your language of words, your baby will feel very much a part of your world. This is called mirroring and is a delightful game for newborns and babies.
- The following research on the development of your baby's brain details the tremendous advantages for our babies when we take the time to talk with them.

New Discoveries on the Development of Your Baby's Brain

Excerpted from Newsweek, *February 1996, Newsweek, Inc. "Your Child's Brain: How Kids are Wired for Music, Math and Emotions", Sharon Begley. All rights reserved. Reprinted with permission.*

A baby's brain is a work in progress, trillions of neurons waiting to be wired into a mind. The experiences of childhood, pioneering research shows, helps form the brain's circuits for music, math, language and emotions.

You hold your newborn so his sky-blue eyes are just inches from the brightly patterned wallpaper. ZZZZt a neuron from his retina makes an electrical connection with one in his brain's visual cortex. You gently touch his palm with a clothespin; he grasps it, drops it, and you return it to him with soft words and a smile. Crackle; neurons from his hand strengthen their connection to those in his sensory-motor cortex. He cries in the night: you feed him, holding his gaze because nature has seen to it that the distance from a parent's crooked elbow to his eyes exactly matches the distance at which a baby focuses. Zap; neurons in the brain's amygdala send pulses of electricity through the circuits that control emotion. You hold him on your lap and talk and neurons from his ears start hardwiring connections to the auditory cortex. And you thought you were just playing with your kid.

When a baby comes into the world her brain is a jumble of neurons, all waiting to be woven into the intricate tapestry of the mind. Some of the neurons have already been hard-wired, like the genes in the fertilized egg, into circuits that command breathing or control heartbeat, regulate body temperature or produce reflexes. But trillions upon trillions more are like the Pentium chips in a computer before the factory preloads the software. They are pure and of almost infinite potential, unprogrammed circuits that might one day compose rap songs and do calculus, erupt in fury and melt in ecstasy. If the neurons are used, they become integrated into the circuitry of the brain by connecting to other neurons: if they are not used, they may die. It is the experiences of childhood, determining which neurons are used, that wire the circuits of the brain as surely as a programmer at a keyboard reconfigures the circuits in a computer. It determines whether the child grows up to be intelligent or dull, fearful or self-assured, articulate or tongue-tied. Early experiences are so powerful, says pediatric neurobiologist Harry Chugani of Wayne State University, that "they can completely change the way a person turns out".

Once wired, there are limits to the brain's ability to create itself. Called "critical periods" they are windows of opportunity that nature flings open, starting before birth, and then slams shut, one by one, with every additional candle on the child's birthday cake. . . Neurobiologists are still at the dawn of understanding exactly which kinds of experiences, or sensory input, wire the brain in which ways. They know a great deal about the circuit for vision. It has a neuron-growth spurt at the age of 2 to 4 months, which corresponds to when babies start to really notice the world, and peaks at 8 months, when each neuron is connected to an astonishing 15,000 neurons. A baby whose eyes are clouded by cataracts from birth will, despite cataract-removal surgery at the age of 2, be forever blind. . . The implications of this new understanding are at once promising and disturbing. They suggest that, with the right input at the right time, almost anything is possible. But they imply, too, that if you miss the window you're playing with a handicap.

The language brain has a learning window from birth to ten years. Circuits in the auditory cortex, representing the sounds that form words, are wired by the age of 1. The more words a child hears by 2, the larger her vocabulary will grow. Hearing problems can impair the ability to match sounds to letters.

What we can do about it: Talk to your child – a lot. If you want her to master a second language introduce it by the age of 10. Protect hearing by treating ear infections promptly. As the basic circuitry is established a baby is primed to turn sounds into words. the more works a child hears, the faster she learns language, according to Janellen Huttenlocher of the University of Chicago. Infants whose mothers spoke to them a lot know 131 more words at 20 months than did babies of more taciturn, or less involved caregivers. At 24 months, the gap had widened to 295 words. It didn't matter which words the caregiver used, monosyllables seemed to work. The sound of words, it seems, builds up neural circuitry that can then absorb more words, much as creating a computer file allows the user to fill it with prose. There is a huge vocabulary to be acquired, says Huttenlocher, and it can only be acquired through repeated exposure to words.

The logical brain has a learning window from birth to 4 years. Circuits for math reside in the brain's cortex, near those for music. Toddlers taught simple concepts, like one and many do better in math. Music lessons may help develop spatial skills.

What we can do about it: Play counting games with a toddler. Have him set the table to learn one to one relations, one plate, one fork per person. Giving preschoolers piano or singing lessons has been shown to increase the children's ability to work mazes, draw geometric figures and copy patterns of two-color blocks. It is suspected that when children exercise cortical neurons by listening to classical music they are also strengthening circuits used for mathematics. Music, says a team of researchers from UC Irvine excites the inherent brain patterns and enhances their use in complex reasoning tasks. Early musical training develops spatial intelligence, the ability to visualize the world accurately and this skill later translates into complex math and engineering skills. "Early music training can also enhance a child's ability to reason," says Irvine physicist Gordon Shaw.

The greatest effect a parent can have on emotions comes through "attunement" or playing back a child's inner feelings. If a baby's squeal of delight at a puppy is met with a smile and hug, if her excitement at seeing a plane overhead is mirrored, circuits for these emotions are reinforced. Apparently, the brain uses the same pathways to generate an emotion as to respond to one. So if an emotion is reciprocated, the electrical and chemical signals that produced it are reinforced. But if emotions are repeatedly met with indifference or a clashing response – those circuits become confused and fail to strengthen. The key here is repeatedly, one dismissive harrumph will not scar a child for life. It is the pattern that counts, and it can be very powerful. In one of Stern's studies, a baby whose mother never matched her level of excitement became extremely passive unable to feel excitement or joy."

The Emotional Development of Your Baby

Your baby's primary emotional development is set quite firmly into place during the first three years, as shown in the studies of Burton White at his Harvard University Project and by other top researchers today. Emotions such as love, joy, excitement, compassion, empathy, bonding and attachment are laid down like tiles upon the floor forming a foundation for your baby's emotional life.

You can help your baby to recognize and acknowledge feelings by mirroring back to them as they occur. Your baby's excitement can become your excitement. Your baby learns empathy when you soothe their cries. Your baby understands compassion when you respond to feeding, changing, and comfort needs. Your baby experiences love as you gaze deeply into each others eyes. Anger and fear seem to need no introduction to your baby and both seem to be permanently installed from day one as a part of the fight or flight instinct.

The best ways to enrich your baby's emotional development are as follows:
1. Hug your baby often.
2. Crawl Baby Crawl – Find ways to let your baby explore the world safely.
3. Always respond to your baby's coos and cries.
4. Sing to your baby.
5. Create discipline by making meals and naps predictable.

A recent television special entitled, *This Is Your Child*, gives a common sense approach to your baby's emotional and intellectual development. For information on this program call 1-888-447-3400. This program can also be accessed on the internet at www.iamyourchild.org.

Playing With Your Baby

Speak to your baby. Tell your baby how big she is growing. Explain what you are doing, where you are going, noises your baby hears, names of things, how things work, as well as names of the people around you. Every time you communicate with your baby, your baby learns a new word or sound of your language. Just as when you are learning a foreign language, you learn much about what someone is communicating with you by words, gestures and tone of voice.

• Play the alphabet game with your baby by sounding out the letters of the alphabet. Start with the sound of A and finish with the sound of zzzzzz.

Your baby will love to hear certain letter sounds like sssss, and will be fascinated to hear the sounds of your language one at a time. Babies love to hear this game over and over and it may win you your first smile.

- When you feel excited, whether about a certain outing you will be taking or an event that is happening show your baby your excitement. Your baby will feel your excitement and will then feel included in what is going on around her.
- When you see that your baby is entranced with something visually, notice it yourself and talk about the item. By observing the behavior of your baby you will begin to build a bridge of communication between the both of you.
- Babies love to dance with you, cheek to cheek, to your favorite music.
- Give your baby a gentle massage over her clothes upon awakening from a nap.
- Smile at your baby whenever you remember and you will have a baby who smiles at you.
- Kiss your baby as often as you like. All babies thrive on love, affection and praise, and most especially when this encouragement comes from you.
- Sit your baby up as much as possible when your baby is alert, this gives your baby a much better view of the world. Make sure you are supporting your newborn's head and neck.
- When your baby is stretching after a nap, gently tug on her arms and legs along with her.
- Bundle up your baby in a blanket and go for a walk around the block. Some babies are calmer and sleep better after some fresh air.
- Play music for your baby whenever possible as music increases the development of your baby's brain. A portable Fisher Price tape recorder is an excellent way to have music in the bath, the kitchen and all around the house and outside. Experiment with different types of music and you will probably find that your baby has quite a sophisticated taste in music and will especially like any music that you enjoy.
- Cuddle up together with your baby on your chest. Have a short nap or just daydream together.
- Play with your baby's arms, legs, toes and fingers.
- Your baby loves to look at bright lights. Go out in the evening after dark for a short walk and look at the stars and street lights.
- Turn the radio up in the car and sing to your baby.
- Make silly faces or silly noises.
- Play pat-a-cake or little piggies with your baby.
- Bring your baby around to different rooms and explain what you are doing. Babies love to play in a basket of freshly dried clothes and they can

help to make that endless chore go more quickly for you.

- The first year with your baby is full of excitement, exploration and exhaustion. Spend as much time as you can down on the floor with your baby and encourage your partner to do so as well. Your baby will show you things you never thought possible. Talk to her, hold her and love her. By the end of that first year, she is ready to pull away and be more independent and it gets progressively harder to cuddle her and just hold her. Once she learns to walk, she wants to move. Enjoy those first few months of closeness because it will never be just that way again.

Play with a Purpose

Excerpted from Gymboree Parent Play Guide *the world's leading play program combining fun, learning, activity and music in an interactive environment for parents and babies. Expect to have just as much fun, or more, as your baby. Developmentally appropriate classes are offered for newborns through five years of age. Gymboree has experience with over 1,000,000 families worldwide in over 375 locations around the world. You can locate a program near you by calling the head office of Gymboree Corporation at 1-415-579-0600 or in the U.S. 1-800-520-PLAY. The* Gymboree Parent Play Guide *is available free of charge by writing to The Gymboree Corporation, Attention:* Parent Play Guide, *700 Airport Boulevard, Suite 200, Burlingame, CA 94010-1912, USA.*

When your child approaches a new physical activity, praise and support him no matter what his level of mastery. Encourage him to try activities again, be close to offer help and support, and applaud his accomplishments enthusiastically. Remember there is no right or wrong way for a child to approach a new physical activity, as long as it is safe! Keep in mind that all activities in this guide are to be done under parental supervision.

When helping children to walk, support them around the torso or hold the back of their clothing. Doing so frees their arms for better balance. This applies to children from early walkers taking their first steps to older children trying a balance beam for the first time.

Make car trips more fun by having several familiar musical tapes handy. Younger children will be soothed by the familiar music, older ones will join in and sing for entertainment.

Enhance every activity you participate in with your child by promoting language development. Talking while dressing and bathing helps even young babies understand the rhythm, flow, use and meanings in language. With older children, name and count objects and colors, identify directions like going up or down and spatial concepts like through, on, over, as you and your child experience these activities.

Maintain eye contact with your child when he is trying a new activity, such as crawling through a tunnel. For instance, place yourself at one end of the tunnel and look through to the child to provide a familiar landmark and friendly encouragement.

For a baby who is about to crawl, place hands under the soles of baby's feet and gently support them while crawling. Let baby push against your hands, rather than you pushing baby. This works especially well when baby is attempting to crawl up a small incline.

Let your children crawl and walk barefooted as much as possible. Doing so strengthens foot muscles and provides tactile stimulation.

Simplify for success. Make sure you are providing play opportunities in which your child can be successful. As she develops self-confidence and mastery of an activity, begin to build in new and more advanced challenges.

Remember, each child develops at his own pace. Encourage your child's curiosity and willingness to test new feats. This will promote self-esteem and build confidence, the most important accomplishment of all!

Practice makes permanent. Remember that children learn through repetition. Activities that they enjoy may be repeated again and again, each time with a little more mastery than the last.

Young children learn by integrating information gathered through their sensory systems. The following play ideas will assist your baby in learning the developmental tasks of balance, motor planning, spatial awareness, and will help to develop your baby's auditory, visual and tactile systems. A play program at Gymboree will show you how to make the most of play with your baby. Most programs feature over forty pieces of gym equipment created especially for babies and crawlers to help you to play safely as well. Here are some parent interactive activities you can use at home:

Place sofa cushion and pillows on the floor. Lay baby on tummy with arms and head over the edge of cushion. Baby can push up with arms in preparation for crawling. Scatter cushion as an obstacle course for baby to crawl over and around.

Using the leaf from your dining room table, set up a slide for baby. Place leaf on the edge of couch or chair for a gentle incline. Make sure it is on carpeting or padding for safety. Supervising carefully, place baby on tummy to slide feet first. Baby can also crawl up the leaf as a ramp.

Fill your big tub with water for baby to sit in and play with a variety of toys. Use various sponges and cloths to wash your baby for different tactile experiences. On a summer morning, place a small tub outside and fill with water. By afternoon, the water will be warm enough for play. Never leave your baby unattended in close proximity to water.

Make baby's first tunnel out of a large box. Lay the box on its side and cut off ends Be sure to remove all staples. Maintain eye contact with baby as you place him inside the tunnel.

Place baby on tummy on top of a ball and gently roll ball in all directions. Older babies may sit upright atop ball. Baby Soccer: Hold child by the trunk and gently swing him to kick ball with his feet. Ball may be kicked to another person or against a wall.

Blow bubbles for babies to watch and to reach. As baby sits up, hold bubble on the end of a wand for him to reach out and pop. A great activity to encourage eye tracking and eye-hand coordination.

Place baby on back on center of small sturdy blanket. With two adults each holding two blanket corners, gently and careful swing baby side to side and head to foot. Lift the blanket up and down for even more fun.

To enhance self awareness, place shatterproof mirrors at floor level so baby can see himself. Play peek a boo by covering the mirror with a scarf.

Stand an inner tube on its side and place baby inside with upper torso resting on tube in crawling position. Baby will push up in preparation for crawling. Place toys and balls within easy reach for baby to play with.

Hide a music box or alarm clock under a blanket. Let baby react to the noise and look for the source of the sound.

Let baby focus on a beam of light and track it on the wall. For more challenge move the light in circles and at a different pace, fast and slow.

Play peek a boo by putting a scarf or cloth over your head. Eventually your baby will experience cause and effect by pulling the scarf off himself.

The Magic of 21

Researchers have long known the magic of 21 in learning a new habit or in releasing an old one. New research is now showing this number is valuable for babies and children as well. If we carefully watch our children at play we notice that they will repeat the exact same activity for an exact number of times. This number is 21 times.

This number correlates directly to the exact number of times an activity needs to be repeated in order to be permanently placed into the neural pathways of the brain. The first pathway is like a line, then a tiny path, then a road, then a two-lane highway, four-lane highway, and finally an expressway into the mind. When the expressway or neural pathway is completed, after 21 times, a myelin coating then covers that pathway making it permanent. The myelin coating speeds conduction of thought whenever that task needs to be repeated. Thus as your baby begins to laboriously open and close that tightly clenched fist it becomes easier and easier with each attempt.

If the baby or child is interrupted before a set pattern of repetitions have occurred in a new learning experience, the pathway will not be completely developed, frustrating the child. To allow the greatest amount of learning to take place it is often best to allow them to decide the exact amount of attempts needed to complete a task. So when you watch your baby in a new play activity, watch for the magic of 21 and you will see the pride and satisfaction in your baby when the task at hand has been successfully completed.

Eye Contact

It takes a few months before your baby will establish direct eye contact with you when you speak. Watch for moving arms and legs to assure you that indeed your baby is listening to you.

Your newborn has perfect vision of twelve to eighteen inches at birth. Just far enough away to see your smiling face as you are feeding or holding your baby. Make sure you have everyone keep their faces back at least 12 inches to avoid overwhelming your baby in the first few months.

Your baby will focus mainly on your hairline and will be memorizing the contrast of your skin and hair. Your baby is using many of her senses to get to know you and your partner besides her vision with her sense of touch, sense of smell, sense of taste, and hearing. Your baby can hear you even though she is not looking directly at you. Don't let it discourage you from talking to your baby as much as you can.

Baby Signs

Baby hand signs are non-verbal gestures taught to allow your baby to communicate with you before she begins to speak. You can easily begin by appreciating the baby signs you are already using naturally such as:

1. Waving Bye-Bye.
2. Nodding head up and down for yes.
3. Shaking head for no.
4. Saying "Shhh" with your fingers across lips for sleeping.
5. Showing empty hands to say all gone.

Other easy signs to help your baby communicate:

6. Hat – Tap the top of your head.
7. Bird – Flap one or both arms.
8. Flower – Sniffing gesture.
9. Fish – Open and close lips making smacking noises.
10. More – Tap the index finger of one hand into opposite palm.

Other signs to connect with your baby's world include:

11. Duck – Keep fingers straight and open and close like a beak.
12. Cat – Stroke the back of your arm with fingers like stroking a cat.
13. Dog – Open your mouth and pant.
14. Bottle/Drink – Put thumb to your lips and tilt your head as if drinking.
15. Eat – Two fingers pressed against lips.

Saying the word along with the sign gives your baby the opportunity to understand either method of communication with you. For more fascinating reading on this ground breaking work with babies read *Baby Signs: How To Talk With Your Baby Before Your Baby Can Talk,* Linda Acredolo, PhD, and Susan Goodwyn, PhD, 1996.

Startle Reflex

When moved abruptly from place to place, your newborn may startle. Pick up your baby slowly and gently, and have others do the same, holding your baby close to your body when you are moving.

When putting your baby down for a nap or onto the change table, keep your hand on your baby for a minute after. If your baby startles, gently press both of baby's arms together with your hands, hold for 30 seconds and gently reassure your baby.

Sneezing

Your baby sneezes to remove the amniotic fluid from her lungs and to blow her nose. This can happen off and on for a few months. Your baby may also have a raspy sound to the breathing from the amniotic fluid as well.

Ear Infections

Research is now showing that liquid can travel into the middle ear while feeding causing ear infections. Liquid is more likely to drain out and away from the ear canal when the baby is fed in a semi-upright position. If you are lying down during breastfeeding simply place your arm under your baby's head to raise the head sufficiently. Keep your baby's head raised above the body for all feedings, especially during the last few moments to avoid this problem. A bottle to bed can also contribute to ear infections and should be avoided.

Multiple ear infections, continual colds and a runny nose could be a sign of a dairy intolerance. Changing to a soy baby formula for a short time will give you an excellent indication if this is the case.

Ear infections that are not treated can cause serious hearing loss for your baby. A middle ear infection can make a baby or child extremely ill very quickly, with high fever and great pain. A doctor should be called immediately if an ear infection is suspected. Treatment, usually with antibiotics will prevent a burst ear drum and possible damage to hearing. The child may be ill without making it obvious that his ear is the cause; this is why a doctor will always examine an ill child's ears even if they do not appear to hurt.

If the ear infection turns out to be mild after being checked by the doctor you have the option of not using antibiotics to heal it. Repeated use of antibiotics can cause a deposit to build up behind the ear drum.

Dehydration

Dehydration in a newborn is cause for alarm. After the first week you will want to see at least six very wet diapers per day. Dehydration usually occurs as a result of vomiting and loose bowels. Signs of dehydration include listlessness, lack of tears, flaccid muscle tone, or being unable to rouse your baby. Always keep an eye on how many wet diapers your baby has during the day as this will let you know how much fluid your baby is ingesting. An extremely dehydrated newborn will show a marked depression on the top portion of her head. If you see any of these danger signs, immediately call your doctor or nearest emergency department.

Dehydration is not the simple drying out that the name suggests. A body that is seriously short of water cannot maintain the complex and delicate balance of chemicals on which its functioning depends. This is why a baby or very young child who has become dehydrated will not instantly be restored by a drink of water. He will need a careful mixture of chemicals and fluid dripped directly into his bloodstream. Diarrhea and/or vomiting, especially if accompanied by fever, makes a baby very liable to dehydration because each episode may deprive his body of more fluid than his last drink put in. The younger the child, the greater this risk. Babies under six months should be seen by a doctor as a matter of urgency.

Eczema

Infantile eczema tends to run in families. There will probably be a close relative susceptible either to eczema or to some other allergic complaint such as hay fever or asthma. Like all allergic conditions it will be made temporarily worse by anything which upsets the child. The vast majority of children outgrow the eczema by the age of three.

The disorder usually begins with bight red scaly and wildly itching patches on the cheeks. There may well be scurf on the scalp and this may lead to bad patches of itchy rash behind the ears. Occasionally the rash spreads to cover large areas of the body, but it is usually concentrated in the moist creases; in the groin, behind the knees, etc. When the eczema is very active, acute inflammation makes the scaly red patches moist. Eczema itches continually and scratching will make the patches sore and may infect them. Your baby is likely to be desperately miserable.

Eczema is a signal that your baby may have an intolerance to dairy as well as an intolerance to certain perfumes and dyes in soaps and laundry detergents. Rather than use any topical treatment for this irritating skin rash look to see what in your baby's environment may be causing this.

The first place to look is at your laundry detergent. Health food stores now stock laundry detergents completely free of phosphates, dyes, chemicals, perfumes and other additives. Take all of your baby's sheets, blankets, clothing, socks, diapers and wash everything again in the new chemical-free detergent. Just by changing your laundry detergent you can often change the symptoms in a few days. You may also want to try a double rinse on your laundry.

If your baby is still showing some sensitivity, you may want to purchase soapless Ecosave Laundry Discs available at health food stores. These disks are good for over 700 loads of laundry and can be used instead of detergent and fabric softener.

Keep bathing to a minimum and bathe your baby in clear water only, using perfume-free soap or shampoo only in the last moments. If you have hard water in your city a Ecosave magnetic washball gives you rainwater softness in the bathwater by simply dropping the magnetic ball into the tub. This ball can be reused forever and has a lifetime guarantee.

You may also want to remove environmental irritants like tobacco smoke or pets from the home.

Buy cotton instead of polyester clothing for your baby.

You can take all dairy products out of your baby's menu and substitute with soy infant formula to see if this is causing a reaction. If you are breastfeeding remove all dairy products from your diet while you are testing for intolerances. You should be able to track down the offending substance within a short while if the case is a food intolerance. Calendula Cream used directly on the rash can be purchased in health food stores will help relieve your baby's discomfort. Eczema often shows up in children before asthma. Removing food and chemical intolerances from your baby's environment can help to forestall or eliminate asthma. See a homeopath for inexpensive creams and lotions to soothe and protect affected areas. Do not use any cortisone based skin creams on your newborn as it will cause permanent thinning of the skin in that area.

Allergies and Food Intolerances

Sometimes a child who is allergic to a certain protein in her food or drink may produce symptoms that seems entirely unrelated to the digestive tract; eczema, for example or asthma or urticaria. Where food or drink leads to symptoms which are clearly digestive, it is often difficult to tell whether the problem is a true allergy or whether it is one of many kinds of intolerance. Many babies are having reactions to cow milk products. If you are finding any reaction to dairy based products switch immediately to a soy infant formula. If breastfeeding you may want to eliminate dairy products from your diet and take calcium supplements. You may need to try a number of different soy products until you find the one that suits your baby best. Never use regular soy milk products or rice milk as a infant formula for the first year as they will not provide adequate nutritional support. You must use a formula specifically designed for an infant for your baby's first year.

Allergic reactions and intolerances to a food product can show up in a variety of ways such as projectile vomiting, continual diaper rash, wheezing, continual runny nose, drowsiness, swollen eyes, darkened circles under the eyes, lethargy or non-stop crying, or any out of the ordinary symptoms that may occur after your baby has eaten.

Rice milk is a great-tasting, easy to digest and nutritional substitute for cow's milk after the first year when your baby is having three solid meals a day. You can ask any grocery or health food store to stock it for you and it is sold under the name of Rice Dream. Safeway now stocks Rice Dream for all their stores across Canada and they often stock it conveniently beside the other milk in the coolers. Rice milk is packed in one-litre cartons and can be stored on your shelf until you need it.

Solid Foods

Everyone has different advice about when to feed baby solids. Most doctors now recommend that your baby should be mainly on breastmilk or formula for the first year. Many mothers begin to supplement with solid foods after the first six months.

- Your baby may go from breastfeeding to rice cereal, to canned baby food to table food. Or your baby may go from breastfeeding straight to drinking from a cup and eating food from the table.
- All food prepared for your baby should have a wet texture as your baby does not have sufficient saliva to swallow dry food.
- Bland, digestible pure rice cereal mixed with breast milk or applesause and water is a good first food.
- Vegetables and fruits should come next. You may wish to start with vegetables first since babies who become accustomed to the sweetness of fruit sometimes turn up their noses at veggies. Sweet potatoes and yams make an excellent first vegetable. Peel and boil and then mash with a fork adding some of the boiled vegetable water. Carrots and peas are also a good first food and can be easily prepared in the same manner.
- Homemade soups are also a great first food. Slightly overcook the soup to make a soft consistency. Adding rice or noodles to the soup gives variety. If you don't have time to start a soup from scratch, start with a can of soup or a bullion cube and water and add fresh vegetables to it as you go along.
- Introduce one new item at a time, a tablespoon each day. Don't be surprised if your baby spits out the first taste. If your baby rejects a new food, wait a few days and then try again. Your baby is learning new textures as well as new tastes.
- Try not to imitate your baby's faces when you are offering new foods.

Often your baby is reacting to the new texture of the food rather than the taste of it.

- Get creative, mashed potatoes, mashed bananas, instant oatmeal, Cheerios, animal cookies and ritz bits when the teeth come in. Then later, canned or homemade soups, frozen peas, fruits, etc. Watch your baby for clues. Your baby will let you know when she is ready for different tastes and textures. Have your baby join the family at the table when you are eating. Her natural curiosity will serve her and you well.
- If you are breastfeeding you may want to make the decision to continue breastfeeding beyond the first year of your baby's life. Should you stop breastfeeding before the first year and then find out that your baby has food intolerances to dairy or soy milks you may find it difficult to find a replacement food.

The Active Baby

If your baby seems more intense, sensitive, perceptive, persistent or energetic than other babies you may be raising a spirited child. Calming activities for this active baby include gentle massage, a soft lullaby, dim lights or a walk in the sunshine. Extended bath times with sponges, basters, plastic containers, favorite toys and dolls is a calming, soothing activity for this baby. Any one of these activities, especially waterplay of any kind, can scheduled on a daily basis to help calm the active baby.

The mother of an active baby also needs time to relax and recharge. Think about having a 20-minute nap instead of doing one more load of laundry when your baby sleeps. Twenty minutes is the exact period of time in which an adult accesses the relaxing alpha state. Any outdoor activity like walking or gardening are good for both the baby and the mother. Reading the book *Raising Your Spirited Child*, Mary S. Kurchinka, 1991 will give you tremendous insight into your child's personality and temperament along with tools to deal with every situation you may encounter raising an active baby and a spirited child.

You and Your Baby – The First Six Months

Excerpted from Your Baby and Child: From Birth to Age Five *by Penelope Leach, 1997.*

One day you will find that you have stopped regarding your baby as a totally unpredictable and therefore rather alarming novelty and have begun instead to think of him as a person with tastes, preferences and characteristics of his own. When that happens you will know that he has moved on from being a "newborn" and has gotten himself settled into life. Nobody can date that moment except you. An easy birth, close satisfactory contact immediately after it, and a good fit between his needs and your expectations will all tend to bring it forward. Postnatal depression, feeding difficulties, or a baby who needs handling in a way that does not come naturally to you will all tend to keep it back. But whether he is settled at two weeks or at two months, that moment will come.

A settled baby is a manageable proposition. You can tell how he likes to be handled even if it is not the way you would choose to handle him. You know what to expect from him even if it is the worst. You know what frightens him even if it is almost everything. Once your baby is settled you know what you are up against. Instead of trying to survive from hour to hour, get through another day, avoid thinking about another week, you can begin to work and plan for reasonable compromises between his needs and those of everyone else.

Your baby will make it increasingly clear that apart from food, his prime need is for people who are his constant caretakers. Your love for him may still be problematic, but the dawn of his attachment to you is a matter of sheer necessity. If he is to survive, he has to attach himself to you and ensure that you take care of him. As these first few weeks pass, his interest in people becomes increasingly obvious. Your face fascinates him. Every time it comes within his short focusing range he studies it intently, from hairline to mouth, finishing by gazing into your eyes. He listens intently to your voice, kicking a little when he hears it, or freezing into immobility as he tries to locate its source. Soon he will turn his eyes and his head to see who is talking. If you pick him up, he stops crying. If you will cuddle and walk him, he remains content. Whatever else he likes or needs, he clearly likes and needs you. You can begin to have some confidence in yourselves as the parents of this new human being.

But in case these settled responses to your devoted care are not enough to keep you caring, the baby has a trump card still to play: smiling. One day he is studying your face in his intent and serious way and he scans down to your mouth and back to your eyes as usual. But as he gazes, his face slowly begins to flower into the small miracle of a wide toothless grin that totally transforms it. For most parents, grandparents and carers, that's it. Few adults can resist a baby's new smiling. Even the most reluctantly dutiful visitors have been known to sneak back to the cribside to try for one more smile all for themselves.

When the baby smiles it looks like love, but he cannot truly love anyone yet because he does not know one person from another. His early smiles are an insurance policy against neglect and for pleasant social attention. The more he smiles and gurgles and waves his fists at people, the more they will smile and talk to him. The more attention people pay him, the more he will respond, tieing them ever closer with his throat-catching grins and his heart-renderingly quivery lower lip. His responses create a self-sustaining circle, his smiles leading to your smiles and yours to more from him.

There is no harm in assuming that these enchanting early smiles are meant for you personally. They soon will be. It is through pleasant social interaction with adults, who find him rewarding and therefore pay him attention, that the baby moves on from being interested in people in general to being able to recognize and attach himself to particular ones. By the time he is around three months old it will be clear that he knows you. He becomes both increasingly sociable and increasingly fussy about whom he will socialize with. He is ready to form a passionate and exclusive emotional tie with somebody and you are elected.

If a baby's mother is available at all most babies select her for this first love. But the blood-tie doesn't automatically qualify you for the privilege. It has to be earned, not just by being your baby's mother but by mothering him. And mothering does not just mean taking physical care of the baby. The love he is forming is not cupboard love rooted in the pleasures of feeding. Babies fall in love with people who mother them emotionally, talking to them, cuddling them, smiling and playing with them. If you had to share your baby's total care with one other person and you handed over all the physical tasks, using your limited time for loving and play, you would keep your prime role in your baby's life. But if you used your time to meet his physical needs, leaving the other person to be his companion and playmate, it would probably be that companionable adult to whom he became most closely attached. Of course your baby needs good physical care. Of course feeding is his greatest pleasure in life and therefore links physical with emotional care, but your baby doesn't just need someone who'll come and feed him when he's hungry, he needs someone to come when he needs company, someone who notices when he smiles and smiles back, who hears when he "talks", listens and replies. Somebody who plays with him and shows him things, brings little bits of the world for him to see. These are the things which really matter to three month babies. These are the things which make for love.

Every baby needs at least one special person to attach himself to and more are better. It is through this first love relationship that he will learn about himself, other people and the world. It is through them that he will experience emotions and learn to cope with them. And it is through this baby love that he will become capable of more grown-up kinds of love; capable, one far-distant day, of giving children of his own the kind of devotion he now needs for himself. Babies who never have a special person, receiving adequate physical care but little emotional response, or being looked after by a succession of caretakers, often do not develop as fast or as far as their innate drive and their potential for personality allow. And the development of babies who are suddenly separated from parenting people is put at risk. But as long as your baby does have at least one special person he can make other people special too. His capacity for love is not rationed any more than yours is. The reverse is true. Love creates love.

If you and your partner are fortunate enough to be able to share your baby's care from the beginning, he will probably respond equally to each of you in total (though differently since you are different people) and his emotional life will be both richer and safer for not being vested in one person along. That does not mean that you will get equal shares of smiles, or cooperation about stopping crying or going to sleep, on any given day, though. The baby who has the luxury of two available parents will often play favorites. Most babies start out most relaxed of all with their birth mothers – perhaps due to long familiarity with their smells, heartbeats and voices, as well as to the bliss of breastfeeding. By four or five months though, fathers, rather especially the father who has not been continually involved in a baby's routine care, may suddenly find himself singled out for favor. When he does come home, or stays home because it is a weekend, his face, his talk and his play strike the baby as fresh and interesting. Because he has not spend the day trying to fit a sufficiency of chores and sanity-preserving adult activities around the baby's needs, he may be able to offer more of the social contact the baby craves.

Once that special relationship is made, sharing your time between the baby and paid outside work will not threaten it or the baby's well being provided that he continues to be – and to feel that he is – your primary concern, and that the care that fills in for yours is enthusiastic and genuinely loving. Sharing your baby's care with your partner, with other relatives and or with a caregiver whom you pay to act like family, is a modern version of the way babies used to be cared for in extended families in the West, and a Western version of the way they still are cared for in much of the developing world. Don't expect those other people to keep your baby on ice for you, though. He must get on with living and loving in your absence, however much you dread him seeing his first snowfall without you or learning to love them best. The snowfall may happen but won't matter (he won't remember this year's anyway); the loving would matter but won't happen. Once babies know their mothers and fathers from everybody else, they go on knowing. And once they love them best, they go on doing that too.

Many women don't want to share their babies with paid work this soon, though, because they passionately enjoy this stage of motherhood. The baby flatters you with his special attentions, making you feel unique, beloved, irreplaceable. He needs you for everything; for adequate physical care but for emotional and intellectual care too: play, toys, help with each successive effort and opportunity to practise each tiny new accomplishment. Whatever the baby becomes able to do, he needs and will want to do it; it is up to you to make it possible for him. Yet despite all this needing, his hour-by-hour care is comparatively easy. He is no longer irrational and incomprehensible as he was when he was newborn, yet he is not awake most of the day and into everything as he will be in the second half of the year. You still get daytime periods of peace and privacy and you can still put the baby on the floor and know that he will be safely there when you next look.

But some women hate it. Instead of taking pleasure in being so much enjoyed and needed, they feel shut in and consumed by the baby's dependence, yearning for at least a little time when the baby needs nothing practical and nothing emotional either. The continual effort of identifying with his feelings, noticing his needs and padding his journey through the passing days makes them feel drained and once they being to feel like that, practical babycare seems easy compared with coping with an infant's loneliness or boredom.

Understanding your own importance is probably the best prevention and the most likely cure. All the vital developments of these months are waiting inside your baby. He has a built-in drive to practise every aspect of being human, from making sounds, using his hands or rolling over, to eating real food or roaring with laughter. But each aspect of his growing up is also in your hands. You can help him develop and learning or you can hinder him by holding yourself aloof. You can keep him happy and busy and learning fast, or leave him to be discontented, bored and learning more slowly.

If you do help him, you and the whole family will gain because the baby will be comparatively cheerful and easy and a pleasure to have around – most of the time. If you refuse to help him, trying to ration your attention, everyone will suffer and you will suffer most of all. The baby will be difficult, fretful and little pleasure to anyone. You will be unhappy because, however much you may resent the fact, your pleasure and his are tied together. If you please him, his happiness will please you and make it easier for you to go on. If you leave him miserable, his misery will depress you and make it more difficult. You may resent his crying; resent the fact that he needs you – again. But ignoring the crying not only condemns him to cry but also condemns you to listen to his crying. So when you try to meet his needs, tune in to him, treat him as he asks to be treated, you not only do it for him, you do it for yourselves, too. You are a family now. You sink or swim together. Loving a baby in this way is the best investment there is. It pays dividends from the very beginning and it goes on paying them for all the years that there are. He is, after all, a brand new human being. You are, after all, his makers and his founders. As you watch and listen to him, think about and adjust yourselves to him, you are laying the foundations of a new member of your own race and of a friendship that can last forever.

Afterword

This is the book I wanted to read when I was pregnant. I hope you have enjoyed this guide and that you found information within these pages to be of value to you. My thanks go out again to the love, support and guidance from the women and mothers aged 16 to 70 who participated in the research for this project.

I am organizing the Women's Education Fund (W.E.F.) to provide childbirth literature and information to women in every community. I believe that it is imperatively important for women of childbearing years to be informed of the natural birth process and what they can do to have a faster and easier labor and delivery. The first challenge for the Women's Education Fund will be to contact television networks to advise on pregnancy and childbirth issues as shown on television. A great deal of information is absorbed through television programming and in matters of pregnancy and childbirth this information needs to be precise and correct. A webpage is also under construction on the internet co-sponsored by Innovative Publishing and the Women's Education Fund to provide critical pregnancy and childbirth information. This webpage can be accessed by using the key words "pregnancy tips" on the internet. If you would like to contribute to this association contact the W.E.F. through Innovative Publishing.

I am continuously amazed at the miracle of life and birth, most especially when I gaze into the eyes of my daughter. Let us respect this miracle. A calm, gentle entry into life is the best gift we can give our children and our mothers. Best wishes to you and your baby.

Recommended Reading List

The purpose of this guidebook is to direct you to the vast resources now available to first-time mothers. We have chosen some of the best publications on pregnancy, childbirth, breastfeeding and newborn care to assist you in designing the birth you wish to have and give you the support to make it happen. Call the Acquisition Librarian at your local library and ask to have these books stocked for yourself and others. You may wish to add some of these books to your personal library to pass on to your next generation.

Birth

Open Season: A Survival Guide for Natural Childbirth and Vaginal Birth After Cesarean, Nancy Wainer Cohen 1991. Everything you need to know about the politics of birth and how to avoid becoming a pawn in the game. This is a must read for every woman – everywhere.

Homebirth

Homebirth: The Essential Guide for Giving Birth Outside of a Hospital, Sheila Kitzinger 1991. A calm reassuring manual for birth by the internationally known childbirth researcher and educator, Sheila Kitzinger.

Childbirth Research

Obstetric Myths Versus Research Realities. Henci Goer, 1995. Finally the truth about the business of obstetrics. Contains thousands of leading new discoveries in the field of childbirth that you need to know about before you have your baby.

Your Emotional Health

Transformation Through Birth, Claudia Panuthos, 1984. A healing, comforting view of your birth process.

Preventing Cesarean Section

Silent Knife: Cesarean Prevention and Vaginal Birth After Cesarean, Nancy Wainer Cohen and Lois J. Estner 1983. The bible for cesarean prevention.

Creating Your Health Team

Take This Book To The Obstetrician With You: A Consumer's Guide to Pregnancy and Childbirth, Karla Morales and Charles B. Inlander, 1991. Shows you how to be an active participant in your reproductive health care and birth experience.

Professional Labor Support

Mothering The Mother: How a Doula Can Help you Have a Shorter, Easier, Faster

Birth, Marshall H. Klaus, MD; John H. Kennell MD; and Phyllis H. Klaus, MEd, CSW, 1993 A gentle way to have your baby whether you choose home or hospital birth.

Preventing Premature Birth

Every Pregnant Woman's Guide to Preventing Premature Birth, Barbara Luke SCD, MPH, RN, RD, 1995. Excellent information to give your baby the best start.

Premature Care

Kangaroo Care: The Best You Can Do To Help Your Pre-Term Infant, Susan M. Ludington-Hoe; Susan K. Golant, 1993. Everything you need to know about nurturing your premature infant.

Care for the Mother

Mothering The New Mother: Your Postpartum Resource Companion, Sally Placksin, 1994. An excellent source book to help you find everything you'll need as a new mother covering Canada and the United States. Also covers the emotional aspects of being a new mother and the real issues of motherhood.

Postnatal Depression

This Isn't What I Expected: Recognizing And Recovering From Depression And Anxiety, Karen R. Mleiman, McS and Valerie D. Raskin MD, 1993. A life-saver if you experience postnatal depression.

Breastfeeding

Breastfeeding Your Baby, Sheila Kitzinger 1995. Beautiful photographs and an excellent introduction into breastfeeding.

The Womanly Art of Breastfeeding, La Leche League International, 1997. The bible of breastfeeding.

Infant & Child Care

Your Baby and Child: From Birth to Age Five, Penelope Leach, 1997. Internationally known child-care expert covers issues from the medical to the mundane with thoroughness and eloquence. Covers the emotional as well as the practical nature of your baby. If you only buy one book on infant and child care buy this one. The completely revised edition will be released in 1997 and is sure to be one of the best books to have on caring for your baby and child.

Newborn Crying

The Self-Calmed Baby: Teach Your Infant To Calm Itself And Curb Crying,

Fussing and Sleeplessness, William A.H. Sammons MD, 1989. The best book available on understanding the psychology of your newborn along with an easy to follow program that will help your baby to stop crying.

Women's Health
Take Charge of Your Body, Dr. Carolyn DeMarco, 7th Edition, 1997. Dr. DeMarco shows us natural, holistic healing treatments for common health problems in an easy-to-read health manual that every woman should keep in her medicine cabinet.

Alternative Health
Alternative Medicine: The Definitive Guide, compiled by The Burton Goldberg Group, 4th Edition 1995. Over 380 leading edge physicians explain their alternative health treatments. Includes natural, holistic health remedies you can use at home.

Parenting
Positive Discipline, Stephen H. Glenn and Jane Nelsen EdD, 1995. A simple, straight-forward guide for effective discipline that respects both the parent and child.

Raising Self-Reliant Children in a Self-Indulgent World: Seven Building Blocks for Developing Capable Young People, Stephen H. Glenn and Jane Nelsen EdD, 1989. A program you can easily put into place to develop capability within your child.

Raising Your Spirited Child: A Guide for Parents Whose Child is More Intense, Sensitive, Perceptive, Persistent, or Energetic, Mary Kurcinka, 1991. Hundreds of practical suggestions and ideas for adapting to a high-spirited child.

Mail-Order Book Stores
Parentbooks, 201 Harbord Street, Toronto, Ontario M5S lHS (416) 537-8334
Birth and Life Book Store, 7001 Alonzo Ave. NW, Seattle, WA 98107 (206) 789-4444

Bibliography

Acredolo, Linda and Susan Goodwyn. *Baby Signs: How to Talk with Your Baby Before Your Baby Can Talk*. Chicago. Comptemporary Books, 1996.

Balaskas, Janet. *Active Birth*. Harvard. Harvard Common Press, 1992.

Balaskas, Janct. *Water Birth*. London. Unwin Hyman, 1990.

Barrington, Eleanor. *Midwifery is Catching*. Toronto. New Canada Publications, 1985.

Bing, Elisabeth. *Six Practical Lessons for an Easier Childbirth*. New York. Bantam, 1981.

Burch, Frances. *Babysense*. New York. St. Martin's Press, 1991.

Burton Goldberg Group. *Alternative Medicine: The Definitive Guide*. Future Medicine Publishing Inc., 1995.

Brewer, Gail Sforza. *Nine Months, Nine Lessons*. New York, Simon & Schuster, 1983.

Carter, Jenny and Therese Duriez. *With Child: Birth Through the Ages*. Edinburgh. Mainstream Publishing, 1986.

Cohen, Nancy Wainer and Lois J. Estner. *Silent Knife: Cesarean Prevention and Vaginal Birth After Cesarean*. New York. Bergin and Garvey, 1984.

DeMarco, Carolyn, MD. *Take Charge of Your Body*. Winlaw, BC. Well Woman Press, 1997.

Eisenberg, Arlene, Heidi Eisenberg Murkoff, and Sandee Eisenberg Hathaway. *What To Expect When You Are Expecting*. New York. Workman Publishing, 1988.

Eisenberg, Arlene, Heidi Eisenberg Murkoff, and Sandee Eisenberg Hathaway. *What To Eat When You Are Expecting*. New York. Workman Publishing, 1986.

Eisenberg, Arlene, Heidi Eisenberg Murkoff, and Sandee Eisenberg Hathaway. *What to Expect the First Year*. New York. Workman Publishing, 1989.

Eisenberg, Arlene, Heidi Eisenberg Murkoff, and Sandee Eisenberg Hathaway. *What to Expect the Toddler Years*. New York. Workman Publishing, 1994.

Gieve, Katherine. *Balancing Acts on Being a Mother*. London. Virago, 1989.

Glenn, Stephen H. and Jane Nelsen EdD. *Raising Self-Reliant Children in a Self-Indulgent World: Seven Building Blocks for Developing Capable Young People*. Rocklin, CA. Prima Publishing, 1989.

Glenn, Stephen H. and Jane Nelsen EdD. *Positive Discipline*. Rocklin, CA. Prima Publishing, 1995.

Goer, Henci. *Obstetric Myths Versus Research Realities*. Westport, CT. Bergin & Garvey, 1995.

Harper, Barbara, RN. *Gentle Birth Choices*. Rochester, Vermont. Healing Arts Press, 1994.

Kitzinger, Sheila. *Breastfeeding Your Baby.* New York. Alfred A. Knopf, 1989.

Kitzinger, Sheila. *Homebirth: The Essential Guide to Giving Birth Outside of a Hospital.* New York. Dorling Kindersley, 1991.

Kitzinger, Sheila. *The Complete Book of Pregnancy & Childbirth.* New York. Knopf, 1996.

Kitzinger, Sheila. *The Crying Baby.* Great Britain. Penguin Books, 1990.

Klaus & Klaus. *The Amazing Newborn.* New York. Addison Wesley 1988.

Klaus & Klaus. *Mothering The Mother: How a Doula Can Help You Have a Shorter, Easier and Healthier Birth.* New York. Addison-Wesley Publishing, 1993.

Kleiman, Karen, R. NSW and Raskin, Valerie D. MD. *This Isn't What I Expected: Recognizing and Recovering from Depression and Anxiety After Childbirth.* New York. Bantam, 1994.

Kurcinka, Mary. *Raising Your Spirited Child: A Guide for Parents Whose Child is More Intense, Sensitive, Perceptive, Persistent or Energetic.* New York. Harper Collins, 1991.

Korte & Scaer. *A Good Birth, A Safe Birth.* New York. Bantam, 1990.

Laird, Suzanne. *Choices in Childcare.* Calgary. Detselig Enterprises, 1992.

Landis. *Checklist for Your New Baby.* New York. Berkley Book, 1993.

La Leche League. *The Womanly Art of Breastfeeding.* New York. New American Library, 1991.

Leach, Penelope. *Your Baby and Child.* New York. Addison-Wesley, 1997.

Leboyer, Frederick. *Birth Without Violence.* New York. Knopf, 1975.

Lichy, Roger & Eileen Herzberg. *The Waterbirth Handbook: A Guide to the Gentle Art of Waterbirthing.* Bath. Gateway Publishing, 1993.

Lieberman, Adrienne. *Easing Labor Pain.* Boston, Mass. Harvard Press, 1992.

Linden, Paula and Susan Gross. *Taking Care of Mommy.* New York. Franklin Watts, 1983.

Ludington-Hoe, Susan M., PhD with Susan Golant. *Kangaroo Care: The Best You Can Do To Help Your Preterm Infant.* New York. Bantam Books, 1993.

Luke, Barbara, ScD, MPH, RN, RD. *Every Pregnant Woman's Guide to Preventing Premature Birth: Reducing the Sixty Proven Risks That Can Lead to Prematurity.* New York. Times Books, 1995.

Machover, Ilana, Angela Drake, and Jonathon Drake. *The Alexander Technique Birth Book.* New York. Sterling Publishing, 1993.

McCartney, Marion CNW and Antonia VanderMeer. *The Midwife's Pregnancy and Childbirth Book: Having Your Baby Your Way.* New York. Henry Holt & Company, 1990.

Morales, Karla and Charles B. Inlander, *Take This Book To The Obstetrician With You*. New York. Addison-Wesley Publishing, 1991.

Morrone, Wenda. *Pregnant While You Work*. New York. Berkley, 1986.

Nechas, Eileen and Denise Foley. *What Do I Do Now?* New York. Fireside, 1992.

Odent, Michel MD. *Birth Reborn*. London. Souvenir, 1994.

Panuthos, Claudia. *Transformation Through Birth*. Mass. Bergin & Garvey, 1984.

Pryor and Pryor. *Nursing Your Baby*. New York. Harper Collins Publishers, 1991.

Ridgeway, Roy. *Caring for Your Unborn Child*. Northamptonshire. Thorsons, 1990.

Rocissano, Lorraine and Jean Grasso Fitzpatrick. *Helping Baby Talk*. New York. Avon Books, 1990.

Rosen, Mortimer and Lillian Thomas. *The Cesarean Myth: Choosing the Best Way to Have Your Baby*. New York. Penguin Books, 1989.

Sammons, William. *The Self-Calmed Baby*. New York. Little Brown & Co., 1989.

Schrotenboer, Kathryn and Joan Solomon Weiss. *Pregnancy Over 35*. New York. Ballentine, 1985.

Sears, William MD and Martha Sears RN. *The Baby Book*. New York. Little Brown & Co., 1993.

Simkin, Penny, Janet Whalley and Ann Keppler. *Pregnancy, Childbirth and the Newborn*. New York. Simon & Schuster, 1991.

Sloane, Philip, Salli Benedict and Melanie Mintzer. *The Complete Pregnancy Workbook*. Ontario. Key Porter Books, 1986.

Smutny, Joan, Kathleen Veenker, and Stephen Veenker. *Your Gifted Child*. New York. Ballentine, 1989.

Ulene, Art and Steven Shelov. *Bringing Out the Best in Your Baby*. New York. Collier Books, 1986.

Unwin, Carol Dix. *Working Mothers*. London. Hyman, 1989.

Verny, Thomas R. *Nurturing the Unborn Child*. New York, Delacorte Press, 1991.

Young, Catherine. *Mother's Favorites*. Toronto, NC Press, 1988.

Young, Catherine. *Mother's Best Secrets*. Toronto, NC Press, 1992.

Index

"Children are the anchors that hold a mother to life."
Sophicles

To Our Readers:

We love our mail. Send in your best practical tips on pregnancy, childbirth, breastfeeding and newborn care. We will publish the best new tips in our next edition, add your name as a contributor, and send you a gift copy of Pregnancy & Childbirth Tips.

For additional copies of *Pregnancy & Childbirth Tips,* send $18.95, plus $3.50 for shipping and handling, payable to Innovative Publishing. Ask about our excellent discounts for organizations and associations using this publication for fund-raising purposes.

Name: _____

Telephone (   ) _____

Address: _____

              _____

Amount Enclosed: $_____ VISA/CHEQUE/MONEY ORDER

Copies Requested: _____

Account #:_____

Signature: _____Exp/Date: _____

Mail To: INNOVATIVE PUBLISHING

             #2755, 349 West Georgia St.
             Vancouver, BC, V6B 3X2
             Email: (pregnancy.tips@shaw.wave.ca)

For media interviews and speaking engagements contact:
Telephone: (403) 271-2576
Fax: (403) 259-4305

> *"Children are the anchors that hold a mother to life."*
> *Sophicles*

To Our Readers:

We love our mail. Send in your best practical tips on pregnancy, childbirth, breastfeeding and newborn care. We will publish the best new tips in our next edition, add your name as a contributor, and send you a gift copy of Pregnancy & Childbirth Tips.

For additional copies of *Pregnancy & Childbirth Tips,* send $18.95, plus $3.50 for shipping and handling, payable to Innovative Publishing. Ask about our excellent discounts for organizations and associations using this publication for fund-raising purposes.

Name: _____

Telephone (   ) _____

Address: _____

_____

Amount Enclosed: $_____ VISA/CHEQUE/MONEY ORDER

Copies Requested: _____

Account #:_____

Signature: _____Exp/Date: _____

Mail To: INNOVATIVE PUBLISHING

        #2755, 349 West Georgia St.
        Vancouver, BC, V6B 3X2
        Email: (pregnancy.tips@shaw.wave.ca)

For media interviews and speaking engagements contact:
Telephone: (403) 271-2576
Fax: (403) 259-4305